HEALTHY PEOPLE

The Surgeon General's Report On
Health Promotion And Disease Prevention

1979

U.S. DEPARTMENT OF HEALTH, EDUCATION, AND WELFARE

Public Health Service
Office of the Assistant Secretary for Health and Surgeon General
DHEW (PHS) Publication No. 79-55071

For sale by the Superintendent of Documents, U.S. Government Printing Office
Washington, D.C. 20402

Stock Number 017-001-00416-2

DEPARTMENT OF HEALTH, EDUCATION, AND WELFARE
WASHINGTON, D.C. 20201

SURGEON GENERAL
OF THE
PUBLIC HEALTH SERVICE

The Honorable Joseph A. Califano, Jr.
Secretary of Health, Education, and Welfare

Dear Mr. Secretary:

I am pleased to transmit herewith the manuscript of the
Surgeon General's Report on Health Promotion and Disease
Prevention.

I believe this will be an important document for the
American people.

Many people and institutions, too numerous to acknowledge,
have provided valuable assistance in preparing this report.
I would particularly like to express appreciation to
Dr. J. Michael McGinnis, Deputy Assistant Secretary for
Health and his staff, and to Dr. David Hamburg, President
of The Institute of Medicine, of the National Academy of
Sciences, for his leadership in mobilizing the resources
of the Institute to provide the accompanying papers which
present documentation for the report.

Sincerely yours,

Julius B. Richmond, M.D.
Assistant Secretary for Health and
Surgeon General

July 1979

We Americans are healthier today than we have ever been.
Our understanding of the causes of health problems has
grown enormously, and with it our ability to prevent and
treat illness and injury.

We have come to take the seemingly miraculous cures of modern
medicine almost for granted. And we tend to forget that our
improved health has come more from preventing disease than
from treating it once it strikes. Our fascination with the
more glamorous "pound of cure" has tended to dazzle us into
ignoring the often more effective "ounce of prevention".

I have long advocated a greater emphasis on preventing illness
and injury by reducing environmental and occupational hazards
and by urging people to choose to lead healthier lives. So I
welcome this Surgeon General's Report on Health Promotion
and Disease Prevention. It sets out a national program
for improving the health of our people -- a program that
relies on prevention along with cure. This program is
ambitious but achievable. It can substantially reduce both
the suffering of our people and the burden on our expensive
system of medical care.

Government, business, labor, schools, and health professions
must all contribute to the prevention of injury and disease.
And all of these efforts must ultimately rely on the individual
decisions of millions of Americans -- decisions to protect
and promote their own good health. Together, we can make
the goals expressed in this report a reality.

Jimmy Carter

THE SECRETARY'S FOREWORD

It gives me pride that virtually my final official act as Secretary of Health, Education, and Welfare is to release this report. For it deals with a subject that has occupied much of my time and even more of my concern over the past two and a half years.

Let us make no mistake about the purpose of this, the first Surgeon General's Report on Health Promotion and Disease Prevention. Its purpose is to encourage a second public health revolution in the history of the United States.

And let us make no mistake about the significance of this document. It represents an emerging consensus among scientists and the health community that the Nation's health strategy must be dramatically recast to emphasize the prevention of disease. That consensus is as important as the consensus announced in 1964 by the first Surgeon General's Report on Smoking and Health—a document now remembered as a watershed.

This Nation's first public health revolution, of course, was the struggle against infectious diseases which spanned the late 19th century and the first half of the 20th century. That revolution has successfully run its course, at least in the United States and the major industrial nations.

Its strategies included major sanitation measures, the development of effective vaccines and mass immunization. So successful was this first revolution that today, only one percent of people who die before age 75 in the United States die from infectious diseases.

In 1900, the leading causes of death were influenza, pneumonia, diphtheria, tuberculosis and gastrointestinal infections. In that year the death rate from these major acute diseases was 580 for every 100,000 people. Today barely 30 people per 100,000 die each year from these diseases.

Remarkable gains in life expectancy—and declines in infant mortality—have occurred since 1900. They were achieved not just by treatment and by curative medicine, but by preventive and health promoting measures: improved sanitation, better nutrition, the pasteurization of milk, and the control of infectious diseases.

The success of that first revolution means that today the pattern of killing and disabling diseases has shifted drastically. While death from the major acute infectious diseases plummeted between 1900 and 1970, the proportion of mortality from major chronic diseases, such as heart disease, cancer and stroke, increased more than 250 percent.

Today cardiovascular disease, including both heart disease and stroke, accounts for roughly half of all deaths. Cancer accounts for another 20 percent. Accidents exact a fearsome toll of death and disability, particularly among young people.

Clearly, the next public health revolution must be aimed at these new killers and cripplers.

And clearly it makes sense in that revolution to emphasize strategies for preventing these afflictions, rather than relying entirely on treating them after they have already struck.

Not to find and employ those strategies would be irresponsible—as irresponsible as it would have been for our predecessors merely to alleviate the ravages of smallpox and polio and cholera, without attempting to eradicate them.

The worldwide eradication of smallpox was achieved not by finding a cure for that disease, but by deploying a vaccine to prevent it. And we are now coming to realize that victory over today's major killers—heart disease, cancer, stroke and the others—must be achieved more by prevention than by cure.

For a number of years, lack of knowledge about the origins of these chronic diseases barred us from developing such preventive strategies.

That is no longer true. And new knowledge from research is steadily increasing our capacity for prevention.

Shortly after I assumed office in 1977, I asked the Surgeon General to begin work on this report. Together, we have worked on it for more than two years.

In addition, we have launched several ambitious disease prevention and health promotion initiatives—most recently a major effort to deal with alcoholism and alcohol abuse.

This book describes, in clear language and in impressive detail, how much we have learned in recent years: about risk factors associated with heart disease and stroke, for example, and about toxic agents which cause cancer.

I can compress what we have learned about the causes of these modern killers in three summarizing sentences:

We are killing ourselves by our own careless habits.

We are killing ourselves by carelessly polluting the environment.

We are killing ourselves by permitting harmful social conditions to persist—conditions like poverty, hunger and ignorance—which destroy health, especially for infants and children.

To know these things gives hope that we can devise new strategies for health. But medical and scientific knowledge do not automatically confer the power to solve the health problems of today.

What is in doubt is whether we have the personal discipline and political will to solve these problems.

Let me dwell first on the matter of individual discipline and will.

This report underscores a point I have made countless times, again and again, in my thirty months as Secretary of Health, Education, and Welfare: "You, the individual, can do more for your own health and well-being than any doctor, any hospital, any drug, any exotic medical device."

Indeed, a wealth of scientific research reveals that the key to whether a person will be healthy or sick, live a long life or die prematurely, can be found in several simple personal habits: one's habits with regard to smoking and drinking; one's habits of diet, sleep and exercise; whether one obeys the speed laws and wears seat belts, and a few other simple measures.

One study found that people who practiced seven of these simple health habits lived, on the average, eleven years longer than those who practiced none of them.

We can see certain signs that millions of Americans are taking this message to heart: a growing national enthusiasm for exercise; signs that more and more people are having their blood pressures checked—and fewer people, as a result, are dying from heart disease and stroke; and signs that cigarette smoking is declining, as more people recognize smoking for what it really is—slow-motion suicide.

But we are a long, long way from the kind of national commitment to good personal health habits that will be necessary to change drastically the statistics about chronic disease in America.

And meanwhile, indulgence in "private" excesses has results that are far from private. Public expenditures for health care that consume eleven cents of every federal tax dollar are only one of those results.

This is only one difficulty we face in establishing a national strategy of disease prevention and health promotion.

Just as no biomedical researcher or group of them can decide for an individual to give up smoking or to eat sensibly, no physician or group of them can achieve alone the political and industrial reforms necessary to safeguard people against toxic chemicals in the workplace.

And certainly no hospital or clinic can cure the poverty and ignorance that foster unattended pregnancies, or overcome the hunger that causes low birth weight babies.

Let us be clear about one fundamental fact: the changes required, if we are to mount a successful public health revolution in the next generation, go far beyond the traditional health care community.

There will be controversy—and there should be—about what role government should play, if any, in urging citizens to give up their pleasurable but damaging habits. But there can be no denying the public consequences of those private habits.

There will be controversy—and there should be—about how much regulation in the name of environmental safety is necessary and desirable. But there can be no denying the growing evidence that some occupational exposures—to asbestos, to radiation, to pesticides like Kepone, for example—can have devastating health consequences.

And of course there will be controversy about welfare, income maintenance programs, food stamps and other efforts to alleviate poverty.

But we simply cannot avoid the fact that if we are to mount a successful second public health revolution, we must deal effectively with deep social problems that destroy health.

This document is properly optimistic about our growing scientific knowledge and about the possibility of setting clear, measurable goals for public health action.

Indeed, one of the most exciting features of this report is that it clearly lists five public health goals which are both measurable and achievable; one major goal for each major age group in our society between now and 1990:

- A 35 percent reduction in infant mortality by then;

- A 20 percent reduction in deaths of children aged one to 14, to fewer than 34 per 100,000;
- A 20 percent reduction of deaths among adolescents and young adults to age 24, to fewer than 93 per 100,000;
- A 25 percent reduction in deaths among the 25 to 64 age group; and
- A major improvement in health, mobility and independence for older people to be achieved largely by reducing by 20 percent the average number of days of illness among this age group.

But while this book is properly optimistic about the possibility of achieving those goals, it is far more cautious and noncommittal about those larger, more difficult questions of individual and political will. And this, too, is proper—for no book can answer those questions. Only the American people—and their leaders—can.

Joseph A. Califano, Jr.
Secretary
Department of Health, Education, and Welfare

July 26, 1979

TABLE OF CONTENTS

LIST OF FIGURES

SECTION I
TOWARD A HEALTHIER AMERICA

CHAPTER 1

INTRODUCTION AND SUMMARY

The health of the American people has never been better.

In this century we have witnessed a remarkable reduction in the life-threatening infectious and communicable diseases.

Today, 75 percent of all deaths in this country are due to degenerative diseases such as heart disease, stroke and cancer (Figure 1-A). Accidents rank as the most frequent cause of death from age one until the early forties. Environmental hazards and behavioral factors also exact an unnecessarily high toll on the health of our people. But we have gained important insights into the prevention of these problems as well.

It is the thesis of this report that further improvements in the health of the American people can and will be achieved—not alone through increased medical care and greater health expenditures—but through a renewed national commitment to efforts designed to prevent disease and to promote health. This report is presented as a guide to insure even greater health for the American people and an improved quality of life for themselves, their children and their children's children.

Americans Today are Healthier Than Ever

Since 1900, the death rate in the United States has been reduced from 17 per 1,000 persons per year to less than nine per 1,000 (Figure 1-B). If mortality rates for certain diseases prevailed today as they did at the turn of the century, almost 400,000 Americans would lose their lives this year to tuberculosis, almost 300,000 to gastroenteritis, 80,000 to diphtheria, and 55,000 to poliomyelitis. Instead, the toll of *all four* diseases will be less than 10,000 lives.

We have seen other impressive gains in health status in the past few years.

- In 1977, a record low of 14 infant deaths per 1,000 live births was achieved.
- Between 1960 and 1975, the difference in infant mortality rates for nonwhites and whites has cut in half.
- Between 1950 and 1977, the mortality rate for children aged one to 14 was halved.
- A baby born in this country today can be expected to live more than 73 years on average, while a baby born in 1900 could be expected to live only 47 years.
- Deaths due to heart disease decreased in the United States by 22 percent between 1968 and 1977.

FIGURE 1-A

DEATHS FOR SELECTED CAUSES AS A PERCENT OF ALL DEATHS: UNITED STATES, SELECTED YEARS, 1900-1977

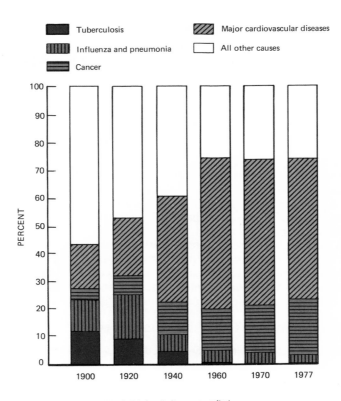

NOTE: 1977 data are provisional; data for all other years are final.

Source: National Center for Health Statistics, Division of Vital Statistics

FIGURE 1B
DEATH RATES BY AGE: UNITED STATES, SELECTED YEARS 1900-1977

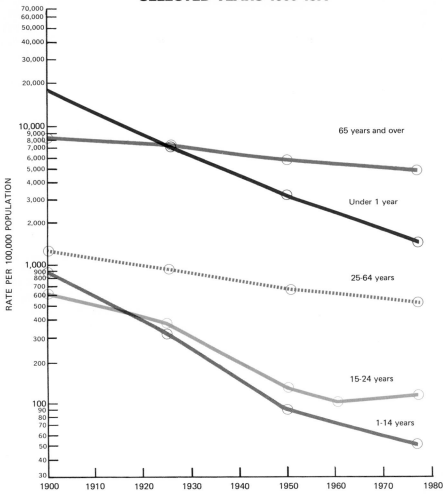

NOTE: 1977 data are provisional, data for all other years are final. Selected years are 1900, 1925, 1950, 1960 (for age group 15-24 years only), and 1977.

SOURCE: National Center for Health Statistics, Division of Vital Statistics.

- During the past decade the expected life span for Americans has increased by 2.7 years. In the previous decade it increased by only one year.

For this, much of the credit must go to earlier efforts at prevention, based on new knowledge which we have obtained through research. Nearly all the gains against the once-great killers—which also included typhoid fever, smallpox, and plague—have come as the result of improvements in sanitation, housing, nutrition, and immunization. These are all important to disease prevention.

But some of the recent gains are due to measures people have taken to help themselves—changes in lifestyles resulting from a growing awareness of the impact of certain habits on health.

Can We Do Better?

To be sure, as a Nation we have been expending large amounts of money for health care.
- From 1960 to 1978 our total spending as a Nation for health care mushroomed from $27 billion to $192 billion.
- In 1960 we spent less than six percent of our GNP on health care. Today, the total is about nine percent. Almost 11 cents of every Federal dollar goes to health expenditures.
- In the years from 1960 to 1978 annual health expenditures increased over 700 percent.

Yet, our 700 percent increase in health spending has not yielded the striking improvements over the last 20 years that we might have hoped for. To a great extent these increased expenditures have been directed to treatment of disease and disability, rather than prevention.

Though, particularly in recent years, we have made strides in prevention, much is yet to be accomplished.

For example, recent figures indicate that we still lag behind several other industrial nations in the health status of our citizens:
- 12 others do better in preventing deaths from cancer;
- 26 others have a lower death rate from circulatory disease;
- 11 others do a better job of keeping babies alive in the first year of life; and
- 14 others have a higher level of life expectancy for men and six others have a higher level for women.

Prevention - An Idea Whose Time Has Come

Clearly, the American people are deeply interested in improving their health. The increased attention now being paid to exercise, nutrition, environmental health and occupational safety testify to their interest and concern with health promotion and disease prevention.

The linked concepts of disease prevention and health promotion are certainly not novel. Ancient Chinese texts discussed ways of life to maintain good health—and in classical Greece, the followers of the gods of medicine associated the healing arts not only with the god Aesculapius but with his two daughters, Panacea and Hygeia. While Panacea was involved with medication of the sick, her sister Hygeia was concerned with living wisely and preserving health.

6

In the modern era, there have been periodic surges of interest leading to major advances in prevention. The sanitary reforms of the latter half of the 19th century and the introduction of effective vaccines in the middle of the 20th century are two examples.

But, during the 1950s and 1960s, concern with the treatment of chronic diseases and lack of knowledge about their causes resulted in a decline in emphasis on prevention.

Now, however, with the growing understanding of causes and risk factors for chronic diseases, the 1980s present new opportunities for major gains.

Prevention is an idea whose time has come. We have the scientific knowledge to begin to formulate recommendations for improved health. And, although the degenerative diseases differ from their infectious disease predecessors in having more—and more complex—causes, it is now clear that many are preventable.

Challenges for Prevention

We are now able to identify some of the major risk factors responsible for most of the premature morbidity and mortality in this country.

Cigarette Smoking

Cigarette smoking is the single most important preventable cause of death. It is clear that cigarette smoking causes most cases of lung cancer—and that fact is underscored by a consistent decline in death rates from lung cancer for former male cigarette smokers who have abstained for 10 years or more.

Cigarette smoking is now also identified as a major factor increasing risk for heart attacks. Even in the absence of other important risk factors for heart disease—such as high blood pressure and elevated serum cholesterol—smoking nearly doubles the risk of heart attack for men.

Though the actual cause of the unprecedented decline in heart disease in the last 10 years is not entirely understood, it is noteworthy that the prevalence of these three risk factors also declined nationally during this same period.

Alcohol and Drugs

Misuse of alcohol and drugs exacts a substantial toll of premature death, illness, and disability.

Alcohol is a factor in more than 10 percent of all deaths in the United States. The proportion of heavy drinkers in the population grew substantially in the 1960s, to reach the highest recorded level since 1850.

Of particular concern is the growth in use of both alcohol and drugs among the Nation's youth.

Problems resulting from these trends are substantial—but preventable. Our ability to deal with them depends, in many ways, more on our skills in mobilizing individuals and groups working together in the schools and communities, than on the efforts of the health care system.

Occupational Risks

Also more widely recognized as threats to health are certain occupational hazards. In fact, it is now estimated that up to 20 percent of total cancer mortality may be associated with these hazards. The true dimensions of the asbestos hazard, for example, have become manifest only after a latency period of perhaps 30 years.

And rubber and plastic workers, as well as workers in some coke oven jobs, are exhibiting significantly higher cancer rates than the general population.

Yet, once these occupational hazards are defined, they can be controlled. Safer materials may be substituted; manufacturing processes may be changed to prevent release of offending agents; hazardous materials can be isolated in enclosures; exhaust methods and other engineering techniques may be used to control the source; special clothing and other protective devices may be used; and efforts can be made to educate and motivate workers and managers to comply with safety procedures.

Injuries

Injuries represent still another area in which the toll of human life is great.

Accidents account for roughly 50 percent of the fatalities for individuals between the ages of 15 to 24. But the highest death rate for accidents occurs among the elderly, whose risk of fatal injury is nearly double that of adolescents and young adults.

In 1977, highway accidents killed 49,000 people and led to 1,800,000 disabling injuries. In 1977, firearms claimed 32,000 lives, and were second only to motor vehicles as a cause of fatal injury.

Falls, burns, poisoning, adverse drug reactions and recreational accidents all accounted for a significant share of accident-related deaths.

Again, the potential to reduce these tragic and avoidable deaths lies less with improved medical care than with better Federal, State, and local actions to foster more careful behavior, and provide safer environments.

Smoking, occupational hazards, alcohol and drug abuse, and injuries are examples of the prominent challenges to prevention, and there are many others.

But the clear message is that much of today's premature death and disability can be avoided.

And the effort need not require vast expenditures of dollars. In fact, modest expenditures can yield high dividends in terms of both lives saved and improvement in the quality of life for our citizens.

A Reordering of our Health Priorities

In 1974, the Government of Canada published *A New Perspective on the Health of Canadians*. It introduced a useful concept which views all causes of death and disease as having four contributing elements:
* inadequacies in the existing health care system;
* behavioral factors or unhealthy lifestyles;

8

- environmental hazards; and
- human biological factors.

Using that framework, a group of American experts developed a method for assessing the relative contributions of each of the elements to many health problems. Analysis in which the method was applied to the 10 leading causes of death in 1976 suggests that perhaps as much as half of U.S. mortality in 1976 was due to unhealthy behavior or lifestyle; 20 percent to environmental factors; 20 percent to human biological factors; and only 10 percent to inadequacies in health care.

Even though these data are approximations, the implications are important. Lifestyle factors should be amenable to change by individuals who understand and are given support in their attempts to change. Many environmental factors can be altered at relatively low costs. Inadequacies in disease treatment should be correctable within the limits of technology and resources as they are identified. Even some biological factors (e.g., genetic disorders) currently beyond effective influence may ultimately yield to scientific discovery. There is cause to believe that further gains can be anticipated.

The larger implication of this analysis is that we need to re-examine our priorities for national health spending.

Currently only four percent of the Federal health dollar is specifically identified for prevention related activities. Yet, it is clear that improvement in the health status of our citizens will not be made predominately through the treatment of disease but rather through its prevention.

This is recognized in the growing consensus about the need for, and value of, disease prevention and health promotion.

Several recent conferences at the national level have been devoted to exploring the opportunities in prevention. Professional organizations in the health sector are re-evaluating the role of prevention in their work.

The President and the Secretary of Health, Education, and Welfare have made strong public endorsements of prevention. And a rapidly growing interest has emerged in the Congress.

The Federal interest is paralleled by great interest in the State health agencies.

There are three overwhelming reasons why a new, strong emphasis on prevention—at all levels of government and by all our citizens—is essential.

First, prevention saves lives.

Second, prevention improves the quality of life.

Finally, it can save dollars in the long run. In an era of runaway health costs, preventive action for health is cost-effective.

Prevention - A Renewed Commitment

In 1964, a Surgeon's General's Report on Smoking and Health was issued. This report pointed to the critical link between cigarette smoking and several fatal or disabling diseases. In 1979, another report was issued based on the knowledge gained from over 24,000 new scientific studies—studies which revealed that smoking is even more dangerous than initially supposed.

In recent years, our knowledge of important prevention measures in other critical areas of health and disease has also increased manyfold.

This, the first Surgeon General's Report on Health Promotion and Disease Prevention, is far broader in scope than the earlier Surgeon General's reports.

It is the product of a comprehensive review of prevention activities by participants from both the public and private sectors. The process has involved scientists, educators, public officials, business and labor representatives, voluntary organizations, and many others.

Preparation of the report was a cooperative effort of the health agencies of the Department of Health, Education, and Welfare, aided by papers from the National Academy of Sciences Institute of Medicine and the 1978 Departmental Task Force on Disease Prevention and Health Promotion. Core papers from both documents are available separately as background papers to this report.

The report's central theme is that the health of this Nation's citizens can be significantly improved through actions individuals can take themselves, and through actions decision makers in the public and private sectors can take to promote a safer and healthier environment for all Americans at home, at work and at play.

For the individual often only modest lifestyle changes are needed to substantially reduce risk for several diseases. And many of the personal decisions required to reduce risk for one disease can reduce it for others.

Within the practical grasp of most Americans are simple measures to enhance the prospects of good health, including:

- elimination of cigarette smoking;
- reduction of alcohol misuse;
- moderate dietary changes to reduce intake of excess calories, fat, salt and sugar;
- moderate exercise;
- periodic screening (at intervals determined by age and sex) for major disorders such as high blood pressure and certain cancers; and
- adherence to speed laws and use of seat belts.

Widespread adoption of these practices could go far to improve the health of our citizens.

Additionally, it is important to emphasize that physical health and mental health are often linked. Both are enhanced through the maintenance of strong family ties, the assistance of supportive friends, and the use of community support systems.

For decision makers in the public and private sectors, a recognition of the relationship between health and the physical environment can lead to actions that can greatly reduce the morbidity and mortality caused by accidents, air, water and food contamination, radiation exposure, excessive noise, occupational hazards, dangerous consumer products and unsafe highway design.

The opportunities are, therefore, great. But if those opportunities are to be captured we must be focused in our efforts.

An important purpose of this report is to enhance both individual and national perspectives on prevention through identification of priorities and specification of measurable goals.

Americans have a deep interest in improving their health. This report is offered to help them achieve that goal.

CHAPTER 2

RISKS TO GOOD HEALTH

Disease and disability are not inevitable events to be experienced equally by all.

Each of us at birth—because of heredity, socioeconomic background of parents, or prenatal exposure—may have some chance of developing a health problem.

But, throughout life, probabilities change depending upon individual experience with risk factors—the environmental and behavioral influences capable of provoking ill health with or without previous predisposition.

Most serious illnesses—such as heart disease and cancer—are related to several factors. And some risk factors—among them, cigarette smoking, poor dietary habits, severe emotional stress— increase probabilities for several illnesses.

Moreover, synergism operates. The combined potential for harm of many risk factors is more than the sum of their individual potentials. They interact, reinforce, even multiply each other.

Asbestos workers, for example, have increased lung cancer risk. Asbestos workers who smoke have 30 times more risk than coworkers who do not smoke—and 90 times more than people who neither smoke nor work with asbestos.

It is the controllability of many risks—and, often, the significance of controlling even only a few—that lies at the heart of disease prevention and health promotion.

Major Risk Categories

Inherited Biological

Heredity determines basic biological characteristics and these may be of a nature to increase risk for certain diseases. Heredity plays a part in susceptibility to some mental disorders, infectious diseases, and common chronic diseases such as certain cancers, heart disease, lung disease, and diabetes—in addition to disorders more generally recognized as inherited, such as hemophilia and sickle cell anemia.

Actually, however, disease usually results from an interaction between genetic endowment and the individual's total environment. And although the relative contributions vary from disease to disease, major risk factors for the common chronic diseases are environmental and behavioral—and, therefore, amenable to change. Even familial tenden-

13

cies toward disease may be explained in part by similarities of environmental and behavioral factors within a family.

Environmental

Evidence is increasing that onset of ill health is strongly linked to influences in physical, social, economic and family environments.

Influences in the physical environment that increase risk include contamination of air, water, and food; workplace hazards; radiation exposure; excessive noise; dangerous consumer products; and unsafe highway design.

Over the past 100 years, man has markedly altered the physical environment. While many changes reflect important progress, new health hazards have come in their wake. The environment has become host to many thousands of synthetic chemicals, with new ones being introduced at an annual rate of about 1,000—and to byproducts of transportation, manufacturing, agriculture and energy production processes.

Factors in the socioeconomic environment which affect health include income level, housing, and employment status. For many reasons, the poor face more and different health risks than people in higher income groups: inadequate medical care with too few preventive services; more hazardous physical environment; greater stress; less education; more unemployment or unsatisfying job frustration; and income inadequate for good nutrition, safe housing, and other basic needs.

Family relationships also constitute an important environmental component for health. Drastic alterations may occur in family circumstances as spouses die or separate, children leave home, or an elderly parent moves in. An abrupt major change in social dynamics can create emotional stress severe enough to trigger serious physical illness or even death. On the other hand, loving family support can contribute to mental and physical well-being and provide a stable, nurturing atmosphere within which children can grow and develop in a healthy manner.

Behavioral

Personal habits play critical roles in the development of many serious diseases and in injuries from violence and automobile accidents.

Many of today's most pressing health problems are related to excesses—of smoking, drinking, faulty nutrition, overuse of medications, fast driving, and relentless pressure to achieve.

In fact, of the 10 leading causes of death in the United States (Figure 2-A), at least seven could be substantially reduced if persons at risk improved just five habits: diet, smoking, lack of exercise, alcohol abuse, and use of antihypertensive medication.

Risk Variability

Because risk factors interact in different ways, population groups which differ because of geographic location, age, and/or socioeconomic strata can experience substantial variability in disease incidence. And in-

14

Figure 2-A

Causes of Death by Life Stages, 1977

AGE GROUPS / PROBLEM	Infants (Under 1) Rank	Rate[1]	Children (1-14) Rank	Rate[2]	Adolescents/ Young Adults (15-24) Rank	Rate[2]	Adults (25-44) Rank	Rate[2]	Adults (45-64) Rank	Rate[2]	Older Adults (Over 65) Rank	Rate[2]	Total Population (all ages) Rank	Rate[2]
Chronic Diseases														
Heart Disease			7	1.1	6	2.5	2	25.5	1	351.0	1	2334.1	1	332.3
Stroke			8	.6	9	1.2	8	6.1[1]	3	52.4	3	658.2	3	84.1
Arteriosclerosis											5	116.5	9	13.3
Bronchitis, Emphysema, & Asthma									10	12.2	8	69.3		
Cancer			3	4.9	5	6.5	1	29.7	2	302.7	2	988.5	2	178.7
Diabetes Mellitus					10	.4	10	2.4	8	17.8	6	100.5	7	15.2
Cirrhosis of the Liver							7	8.6	4	39.2	9	36.7	8	14.3
Infectious Diseases														
Influenza and Pneumonia	5	50.6	6	1.5	8	1.3	9	3.0	9	15.3	4	169.7	5	23.7
Meningitis	6	32.7	8	.6										
Septicemia														
Trauma														
Accidents														
Motor vehicle accidents	7	27.7	2	9.0	1	44.1	3	23.1	7	18.3	10	24.5	6	22.9
All other accidents			1	10.8	2	18.4	4	18.5	5	25.5	7	78.1	4	24.8
Suicide			10	.4	3	13.6	5	17.3	6	19.1			9	13.3
Homicide			5	1.6	4	12.7	6	15.6						
Developmental Problems														
Immaturity associated	1	407.7												
Birth-associated	2	294.4												
Congenital birth defects	3	253.1	4	3.6	7	1.6								
Sudden infant deaths	4	142.8												
All causes		1412.1		43.1		117.1		182.5		1,000.0		5288.1		878.1

[1] Rate per 100,000 live births.

[2] Rate per 100,000 population in specified group.

Source: Based on data from the National Center for Health Statistics, Division of Vital Statistics

15

vestigations of the variability can provide important clues about the extent to which major causes of disease and death may be preventable.

Contrasts between different groups within the United States will be discussed throughout Section II. Here, it is interesting to note some of the striking influences which international variations in habits and environs can have.

For example, an American man, compared to a Japanese man of the same age, is at 1.5 times higher risk of death from all causes, five times higher for death from heart disease, and four times higher for death from lung cancer. And for breast cancer, the death rate for American women is four times as great as for Japanese women. On the other hand, a Japanese man is eight times as likely to die from stomach cancer as his American counterpart. Other Western countries such as England and Wales, Sweden, and Canada have experiences generally paralleling our own although rates vary somewhat from country to country.

The importance of environment and cultural habits, rather than heredity alone, is suggested by studies of Japanese citizens who have moved to the United States. They indicate that, with respect to cardiovascular disease and cancer, families who migrate tend to assume the disease patterns of their adopted country.

Age-Related Risks

From infancy to old age, staying healthy is an ever-changing task. The diseases that affect young children are not, for the most part, major problems for adolescents. From adolescence through early adulthood, accidents and violence take the largest toll. And these are superseded a few decades later by chronic illness—heart disease, stroke and cancer. Figure 2-A depicts major causes of death by life stages.

In one respect, this age orientation is misleading. Although heart disease, stroke, and cancer are commonly regarded as adult health problems, their roots—and, indeed, the roots of many adult chronic diseases—may be found in early life. Early eating patterns, exercise habits, and exposure to cancer-causing substances all can affect the likelihood of developing disease many years later. Some studies have found high blood pressure and high blood levels of cholesterol in many American children. The presence of two such potent risk factors for heart disease and stroke at early ages points to the need to regard health promotion and disease prevention as lifelong concerns.

At each stage of life, different steps can be taken to maximize well-being—and the health goals described in the next section deal with the major health problems of each group.*

---

* The Nation's leading health problems are not only those which cause death. Other significant conditions—such as mental illness, arthritis, learning disorders, and childhood infectious diseases—provoke considerable sickness, disability, suffering, and economic loss. These problems are considered in this report—but, for overview purposes, the leading causes of death provide useful indications of some of the prominent risk factors faced by each age group.

Assessing Risk

Risk estimates are derived by comparing the frequency of deaths, illnesses or injuries from a specific cause in a group having some specific trait or risk factor, with the frequency in another group not having that trait, or in the population as a whole.

Some diseases may occur more frequently in a small population group—for example, a rare type of liver cancer among workers handling vinyl chloride. Such a high risk group, of course, is not difficult to identify although many deaths may occur before the disease cause is clearly established.

But increases in more common diseases not confined to isolated population groups may be much more difficult to attribute to a specific cause. For example, after cigarette smoking was widely adopted, lung cancer rates began to increase dramatically, not immediately but after about a 20-year interval. Because of the large numbers of diverse people and the long interval involved, many theories had to be considered before the direct link between cigarette smoking and lung cancer was firmly established.

The presence of a risk factor need not inevitably presage disease or death. But those events can arise from the cumulative effect of adverse impacts on health. The chain of events may be short, as in a highway accident, or long and complex, as in the development of coronary artery disease and the heart attack which may follow.

Some diseases may involve a single significant risk, such as lack of immunization. Others involve many contributing factors. Those associated with coronary artery disease, for example, include heredity, diet, smoking, uncontrolled hypertension, overweight, lack of exercise, stress, and possibly other unknown factors.

The Role of the Individual

Because there are limits to what medical care can presently do for those already sick or injured, people clearly need to make a greater effort to reduce their risk of incurring avoidable diseases and injuries.

This is not to suggest that individuals have complete control and are totally responsible for their own health status. For example, although socioeconomic factors are powerful determinants, individuals have limited control over them. Nor can they readily decrease many environmental risks. The role of the individual in bringing about environmental change is usually restricted to that of the concerned citizen applying pressure at key points in the system or process. But the individual must rely in large part on the efforts of public health officials and others to reduce hazards.

People must make personal lifestyle choices, too, in the context of a society that glamorizes many hazardous behaviors through advertising and the mass media. Moreover, our society continues to support industries producing unhealthful products, enacts and enforces unevenly laws against behaviors such as driving while intoxicated, and offers ambiguous messages about the kinds of behavior that are advisable.

17

Finally, although people can take many actions to reduce risk of disease and injury through changes in personal behavior, the health consequences are seldom visible in the short run. Even when the individual knows that a habit such as eating excessive amounts of high-calorie, fatty food is not good, available options may be limited. And some habits such as alcohol abuse and smoking may have become addictive.

To imply, therefore, that personal behavior choices are entirely within the power of the individual is misleading. Yet, even awareness of risk factors difficult or impossible to change may prompt people to make an extra effort to reduce risks more directly under their control and thus lessen overall risk of disease and injury. Healthy behavior, including judicious use of preventive health care services, is a significant area of individual responsibility for both personal and family health.

The following sections of this report will clarify the role of various risk factors in disease and disability.

SECTION II - HEALTH GOALS

FIVE NATIONAL GOALS

What should—and reasonably can—be our national goals for health promotion and disease prevention?

They must be concerned with the major health problems and the associated—and preventable—risks for them at each of the principal stages of life: infancy . . childhood . . adolescence and young adulthood . . adulthood . . and older adulthood.

This section examines those problems and risks and presents specific, quantified goals for each stage.

They are realistic objectives—based upon our own recent mortality trends for each age group, the rates achieved in other countries with resources similar to our own, and the very great likelihood that a reasonable, affordable effort can make the goals achievable.

CHAPTER 3

HEALTHY INFANTS

> **Goal:** To continue to improve infant health, and, by 1990, to reduce infant mortality by at least 35 percent, to fewer than nine deaths per 1,000 live births.

Much has happened in recent years to make life safer for babies. The infant mortality rate now is only about one-eighth of what it was during the first two decades of the century (Figure 3-A) thanks to better nutrition and housing, and improved prenatal, obstetrical, and pediatric care. In 1977, a record low of 14 infant deaths per 1,000 live births was achieved, a seven percent decrease from the previous year.

Yet, despite the progress, the first year of life remains the most hazardous period until age 65, and black infants are nearly twice as likely to die before their first birthdays as white infants. The death rate in 1977 for black infants (24 per 1,000 live births) is about the same as that for white infants 25 years ago.

Additional gains are clearly attainable. Sweden, which has the lowest rate of infant deaths, averages nine per 1,000 live births (Figure 3-B). If present trends in the United States continue, our rate should drop below 12 in 1982, and new preventive efforts could allow us to reach the goal of nine by 1990.

The two principal threats to infant survival and good health are low birth weight and congenital disorders including birth defects (Figure 3-C). Accordingly, the two achievements which would most significantly improve the health record of infants would be a reduction in the number of low birth weight infants and a reduction in the number born with birth defects.

Other significant health problems include birth injuries, accidents, and the sudden infant death syndrome which may be the leading cause of death of infants older than one month.

But not all health problems are reflected in mortality and morbidity figures. It is also important to foster early detection of developmental disorders during the first year of life to maximize the benefits of care. And the first year is a significant period for laying the foundation for sound mental health through the promotion of loving relationships between parents and child.

Subgoal: Reducing the Number of Low Birth Weight Infants

Low birth weight is the greatest single hazard for infants, increasing vulnerability to developmental problems—and to death.

FIGURE 3-A
INFANT MORTALITY RATES: UNITED STATES, SELECTED YEARS 1915-1977

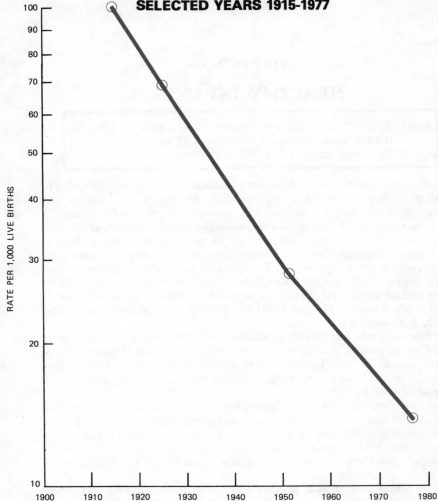

NOTE: 1977 data are provisional; data for all other years are final. Selected years are 1915, 1925, 1950, 1977.

Source: National Center for Health Statistics, Division of Vital Statistics.

22

FIGURE 3-B
INFANT MORTALITY RATES: SELECTED COUNTRIES, 1975

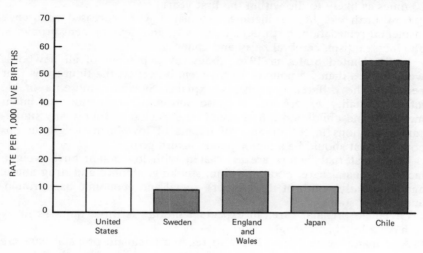

NOTE: The most recent year of data for Chile is 1971.

Sources: United States, National Center for Health Statistics, Division of Vital Statistics; other countries, United Nations.

FIGURE 3-C
MAJOR CAUSES OF INFANT MORTALITY:
UNITED STATES, 1976

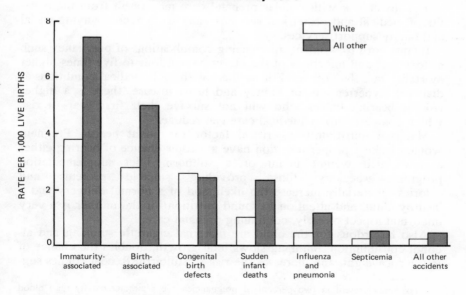

Source: Based on data from the National Center for Health Statistics, Division of Vital Statistics.

Of all infant deaths, two-thirds occur in those weighing less than 5.5 pounds (2500 grams) at birth. Infants below this weight are more than 20 times as likely to die within the first year.

Low birth weight is sometimes associated with increased occurence of mental retardation, birth defects, growth and development problems, blindness, autism, cerebral palsy and epilepsy.

In the United States in 1976, about seven percent of all newborns weighed less than 5.5 pounds. In Sweden, however, the figure was four percent. The difference probably explains Sweden's more favorable infant mortality experience. Because substantial reductions in infant mortality and childhood illness could be expected to follow any significant reductions in the number of infants of low birth weight in this country, that should be a major public health goal.

Many maternal factors are associated with low infant birth weight: lack of prenatal care, poor nutrition, smoking, alcohol and drug abuse, age (especially youth of the mother), social and economic background, and marital status.

Given no prenatal care, an expectant mother is three times as likely to have a low birth weight child.

And many women least likely to receive adequate prenatal care are those most likely to have other risk factors working against them.

Women from certain minority groups are half as likely as white women to receive the minimum of prenatal care recommended by the American College of Obstetrics and Gynecology. About 70 percent of expectant mothers under age 15 receive no care during the first months of pregnancy, the period most important to fetal development; 25 percent of their babies are premature, a rate three times that for older mothers.

The lower risk with regular prenatal care may result from the benefits of medical and obstetrical services—and from accompanying social and family support services.

Infants born to women experiencing complications of pregnancy such as toxemia* and infections of the uterus have a four to five times higher mortality rate than others. For mothers with such medical conditions as diabetes, hypertension, or kidney and heart disease, there is a higher risk of bearing babies who will not survive their first year—a risk which competent early medical care can reduce.

Maternal nutrition is a critical factor for infant health. Pregnant women lacking proper nutrition have a greater chance of bearing either a low birth weight infant or a stillborn. Diet supplementation programs—especially those providing suitable proteins and calories—materially increase the likelihood of a normal delivery and a healthy child, and attention to sound nutrition for the mother is a very important aspect of early, continuing prenatal care.

Also hazardous for the child are maternal cigarette smoking and alcohol consumption. Smoking slows fetal growth, doubles the chance of low birth weight, and increases the risk of stillbirth. Recent studies sug-

---

* Toxemia—present in two percent of pregnancies— is characterized by high blood pressure, tissue swelling, headaches, and protein in the urine. It can provoke convulsions and coma in the mother, death for the fetus.

gest that smoking may be a significant contributing factor in 20 to 40 percent of low weight infants born in the United States and Canada. Studies also indicate that infants of mothers regularly consuming large amounts of alcohol may suffer from low birth weight, birth defects, and/or mental retardation. Clearly, both previously developed habits need careful attention during pregnancy.

Maternal age is another determinant of infant health. Infants of mothers aged 35 and older have greater risk of birth defects. Those of teenage mothers are twice as likely as others to be of low birth weight. And subsequent pregnancies during adolescence are at even higher risk for complications. Family planning services, therefore, are important—and, for pregnant adolescents, good prenatal care, which can improve the outcome, is receiving increased emphasis in many communities.

Racial and socioeconomic groups show great disparity in low birth weight frequency. Not only is infant mortality nearly twice as high for blacks as for whites, prematurity and low birth weight are also twice as common for blacks and some other minorities.

Evidence indicates that the racial differential is associated with corresponding socioeconomic differences. Analyses of birth weight distribution according to socioeconomic status among homogeneous ethnic populations reveal a clear relationship between birth weight and social class; the birth weight of black infants of higher socioeconomic status is comparable to that of whites.

Marital status is another important factor. In 1975, the risk of having a low birth weight infant was twice as great for unmarried as for married women—at least partly because the unmarried are less likely to receive adequate prenatal care.

Although further research can help define more precisely the relationship between all these factors and low birth weight and infant mortality, we have clear indications of measures which can be taken now to reduce the risks. Chapter 8 is devoted to those measures.

Subgoal: Reducing the Number of Birth Defects

Birth defects include congenital physical anomalies, mental retardation, and genetic diseases. Many present immediate serious hazards to infants. Many others, if not diagnosed and treated immediately after birth or during the first year of life, can affect health and well-being in later years.

Birth defects are responsible for one-sixth of all infant deaths. They are the second leading cause of death for children one to four years old, and the third leading cause for those five to 14 years old.

Nearly one-third of all hospitalized children are admitted because of genetically determined or influenced disorders which often result in long-term economic and social strains for affected families.

Approximately two to three percent of infants have a serious birth defect identified within the first weeks of life—and five to 10 percent of these are fatal. Those most likely to be lethal include malformations of brain and spine, congenital heart defects, and combinations of several malformations.

In about one-fourth of birth defects, the cause is thought to be purely genetic; in one-tenth, purely environmental. In the remaining two-thirds, the cause is unknown. Interaction between genetic and environmental factors is an important concept guiding substantial research in this area.

Given current knowledge, many birth defects cannot be prevented. But many can be. Identifiable environmental hazards can be reduced. Carrier identification, amniocentesis, and neonatal screening procedures (Chapter 8) can aid in detecting some genetic disorders before, during, and after pregnancy.

Inherited Factors

Although some 2,000 genetic disorders are known, fewer than 20 are responsible for most genetic disease in this country.

Five types cause most of the illness and death:

Down syndrome. One of the best known genetic disorders, Down syndrome is associated with the presence of an extra chromosome, and occurs in about one of every 1,000 births. It causes physical defects which require lifelong care, and is responsible for 15 to 30 percent of the severe mental retardation in children living to age 10.

The risk of having a Down syndrome child increases with maternal age, especially after 35; at least one-fourth of the 3,000 infants with the syndrome born each year are those of women 35 or older. Recent research has shown that the father, rather than mother, contributes the extra chromosome in about one-fourth of all cases.

Down syndrome can be detected by sampling intrauterine fluid through amniocentesis but the procedure currently is being performed for only about 10 percent of the 150,000 women aged 35 and older who become pregnant in any one year. The advisability of having amniocentesis depends upon individual circumstances and should be discussed with a physician.

Severe brain and spinal cord (neural tube) defects. Neural tube defects not only occur more frequently than Down syndrome but also result in more deaths within the first month of life.

Characterized by lack of development of parts of the central nervous system or its skeletal protection, neural tube defects include spina bifida (a vertebral column defect) and anencephaly (very small head and brain). The defects occur in about two of every 1,000 infants, half of whom die in the newborn period. In addition to amniocentesis, a maternal blood screening test for a substance called alpha-fetoprotein can detect pregnancies at risk for neural tube defects.

Risk for neural tube defects is 2.5 times greater for whites than other racial groups. At greatest risk are families with previous history of the defects or with an affected child; genetic counseling is recommended for them.

Defects related to particular ethnic groups. These include Tay-Sachs disease, sickle cell anemia, and cystic fibrosis.

Tay-Sachs disease is 100 times more frequent among Jewish families of Ashkenazi (Eastern European) descent than in the general population. Although children with the disease appear normal at birth, they die by age five as a result of severe mental retardation and progressive neurologic deterioration. The disease is caused by accumulation of a fatty substance in the brain. Because the responsible gene is recessive, Tay-Sachs disease occurs only when both parents carry the gene. Each prospective child then has a 25 percent chance of developing the disease. Fortunately, a carrier detection screening test is available to identify an at-risk couple before pregnancy.

Sickle cell anemia is the most common serious genetic disease among blacks. About 1,000 infants each year are born with sickle cell disease in which red blood cells are damaged because of altered stability of their hemoglobin content. Although no mental retardation is associated with sickle cell disease, it is a serious condition leading to years of pain, discomfort, and even death from complications. Specific treatment has yet to be found.

Cystic fibrosis occurs primarily among whites in about one of every 2,000 births, affecting 1,500 infants a year. In the disease, abnormal production of mucus leads to chronic lung obstruction and disability during childhood and early adult life. The disease can also affect the pancreas, liver, and intestines. In 1976, it caused the death of twice as many infants as tetanus, whooping cough, syphilis and rubella combined. Although there is no specific cure, there have been many advances in caring for patients so that, if they survive through infancy, many now reach adult life.

Sex-linked defects. These congenital disorders affect the sons of mothers who carry an abnormal X chromosome. Hemophilia and muscular dystrophy are two prominent examples. The bleeding disorder, hemophilia, is due to deficiencies in the clotting mechanism of the blood. In muscular dystrophy, muscle is replaced by fat, leading to gradual muscular weakness and wasting.

Metabolic disorders. The most widely known of this group—and the one for which infants are most frequently tested—is PKU (phenylketonuria). It involves a genetic liver enzyme deficiency which allows an amino acid to accumulate abnormally, impairing brain function and leading to increasingly severe mental retardation later in childhood. PKU, which occurs in one of every 15,000 births, can be treated with special diet that compensates for the enzyme deficiency.

Cogenital hypothyroidism (cretinism) is a more common metabolic disorder capable of causing mental retardation. Some cases result from genetic predisposition but others may be the result of circumstances (e.g. maternal iodine deficiency) occurring during fetal development. About 600 infants a year—one per 5,000 births—are affected, but early detection and prompt treatment with thyroid medication in the first weeks of life can prevent the retardation.

The availability of specific tests for both PKU and congenital hypothyroidism has prompted States to consider requiring both for each newborn. Even though the number of affected babies detected will be small, the benefits of early diagnosis and treatment for the affected babies can be profound.

Birth defects can result from exposure of the fetus to infectious or toxic agents during pregnancy, especially during the first three months (first trimester).

Infections. Rubella (German measles), when it affects a mother during the first trimester, can lead to congenital malformations as well as still-birth and miscarriage.

The greatest risk occurs when most women may not even be aware of being pregnant. The likelihood of rubella-induced malformations is approximately 25 percent during the first three months, after which it begins to decline substantially. The most serious problems for the fetus include blood disorders, heart defects, cataracts or other eye defects, deafness, and mild to profound mental retardation.

For prospective mothers who have not been exposed to rubella, vaccination prior to pregnancy can help prevent all of the problems for the fetus.

Radiation and chemicals in the workplace. These environmental factors have their greatest potential for harm during the early weeks of fetal development—again, often before a woman realizes that she is pregnant. And they remain hazards throughout pregnancy. High doses of ionizing radiation *in utero* not only can increase risk of fetal malformation, there is suggestive evidence of increased risk of subsequent leukemia and other childhood cancers. To reduce risks, protective measures should be taken to help pregnant women avoid unnecessary exposure.

Drugs. A broad range of medications, including some seemingly innocuous over-the-counter preparations, may harm the fetus.

A now-classic example of drug hazard is the epidemic several years ago of birth defects caused by maternal use of thalidomide. Taken as a mild sedative and sleeping aid, thalidomide led to developmental defects, particularly of the limbs, in approximately 35 percent of infants of mothers using it. Throughout the world, an estimated 10,000 deformed infants were born. Thalidomide was on the European market approximately five years before the problem was identified and the product removed, but it was never approved for use in the United States.

Other drugs known to cause birth defects include some hormones such as DES (diethylstilbestrol), as well as certain anti-cancer and anti-convulsant agents. DES taken by mothers during pregnancy has been linked to vaginal cancer development in daughters during adolescence and early adulthood.

Among drugs currently under study for possible birth defect potential are warfarin, diphenylhydantoin, trimethadione, and lithium. Some women need these drugs for serious problems such as post-rheumatic heart disease, seizures, and severe mental disturbances. Also under investigation are some drugs used during childbirth which may have detrimental effects on the child's central nervous system.

It must be emphasized to the public—and perhaps to some physicians—that exposure to any drug should be avoided at any time during pregnancy, but especially during the first trimester, unless there are overriding medical considerations to use a drug for the mother's health.

Alcohol. The incidence of alcohol-induced birth defects is now estimated to be one for every 100 women consuming more than one ounce
of alcohol daily in early pregnancy. The fetal alcohol syndrome therefore accounts for the occurrence of approximately one birth defect in
every 5,000 births in the United States.

Affected infants are often of low birth weight, mentally retarded, and
may have behavioral, facial, limb, genital, cardiac and neurological abnormalities.

The risk and degree of abnormality increases with increased alcohol
consumption. According to a Boston City Hospital study of infants
born to heavy drinkers (average 10 drinks a day), 29 percent had congenital defects compared to 14 percent for moderate drinkers and only
eight percent among nondrinkers. Furthermore, 71 percent of infants
born to women who consumed more than 10 drinks daily had detectable physical and developmental abnormalities.

Safe alcohol consumption levels during pregnancy have yet to be determined. But, in view of the association between high levels and fetal
abnormalities, women who are pregnant or think they might be should
be encouraged to use caution. And women alcoholics, until treated effectively for their addiction, should be encouraged by public information programs and by direct counseling to avoid conception.

Other Important Problems

Several other problems with major impact on infant health are noted
in Figure 3-C.

Injuries at Birth

Birth injuries, difficult labor, and other conditions causing lack of
adequate oxygen for the infant are among the leading reasons for newborn deaths.

Although most pregnant women experience normal childbirth, complications may occur during labor and delivery. Some—such as small
pelvic cavity—can be detected in advance, during prenatal care.

Others unidentifiable beforehand require prompt management. They
include hemorrhaging from the site of attachment of the placenta (after-
birth); abnormal placental location; abnormal fetal position; premature
membrane rupture; multiple births; sudden appearance or exacerbation
of toxemia; and sudden intensification of a known medical problem
such as heart disease or diabetes.

Sudden Infant Death

Certain babies, without apparent cause or warning, suddenly stop
breathing and die, even after apparently uncomplicated pregnancy and
birth.

This unexplained event, called the sudden infant death syndrome, is
believed by some authorities to be the leading cause of death for babies
older than one month.

Recently evidence has been accumulating that abnormal sleep patterns with increased risk of breathing interruptions (apnea) may be associated with the unexpected deaths. A variety of factors, such as prematurity and maternal smoking, are emerging as possible contributors to increased risk for sudden infant death, but there is a need to learn more.

Extensive research now under way should refine our ability to identify high risk infants and effectively prevent their deaths.

Accidents

More than 1,100 infants died in accidents in 1977. The principal causes were suffocation from inhalation and ingestion of food or other objects, motor vehicle accidents, and fires. Many deaths reflect failure to anticipate and protect against situations hazardous for developing infants. Child abuse may also account for some deaths.

Inadequate Diets and Parental Inadequacy

Although they are not major causes of death, problems related to infant care have significant impact on infant health.

Even in a society of considerable affluence, many infants are not receiving appropriate diets and suffer from deficiencies of nutrients needed for development. Frequently, it is overnutrition rather than undernutrition which is the problem setting the stage for obesity later in life.

Recognition of the extent to which parental attitudes are important to a child's development— and, with it, the need to bring parents and babies together psychologically—is receiving increasing attention.

Even when an infant must be kept in the hospital because of low birth weight, early contact between parents and child may be helpful to a good start in life and sound emotional development. Breast feeding is to be encouraged not only for its nutritional benefits but also for the contribution it can make to psychological development.

The fact is that growth of a "sense of trust" has been identified as a significant aspect of healthy infancy. Intimate, enjoyable care for babies fosters that growth and the building of sound emotional and mental health.

Moreover, recently, there has been growing recognition that certain disorders occur when there is neglect or inappropriate care for an infant. One is "failure to thrive" or developmental attrition— with the child losing ability to progress normally to more complex activities such as standing, walking, talking, and learning. Other disorders linked to neglect or inappropriate care include abnormalities in eating and digestive functions, sleep disorders, and disturbances in other activities.

• • • •

All of these problems underscore the need for regular medical care during the prenatal period and early months of infancy. Such care should be sensitively designed to enhance the relationship between parents and child as well as to ensure sound nutrition, appropriate immunizations, and early detection and treatment of any developmental problems.

As programs have expanded to provide better services to pregnant women and newborn babies, the health of American infants has steadily improved. These recent gains to infant health are indeed heartening.

Moreover, more can be done. To a greater extent than ever before, we have a clearer understanding of the factors important to ensuring healthy infants.

Section III discusses in greater detail the actions we can take.

CHAPTER 4

HEALTHY CHILDREN

Goal: To improve child health, foster optimal childhood development, and, by 1990, reduce deaths among children ages one to 14 years by at least 20 percent, to fewer than 34 per 100,000.

The health of American children is better than ever before. The childhood mortality rate now is far below what it was in 1900 when 870 of every 100,000 children ages one to 14 years died annually (Figure 4-A). Then, the principal causes of death were infectious diseases—and, although they still are responsible for some illness and death, their threat has been greatly reduced through improved sanitation, nutrition and housing, as well as use of vaccines and antibiotics.

By 1925, the death rate for children had fallen to 330 per 100,000; by 1950, to 90; and by 1977, to 43.

Yet, there is cause for concern.

- Black American children have a 30 percent higher mortality rate.
- For all our children at ages one to 14 the death rate is still slightly higher than for those in some other countries (Figure 4-B).
- And our rate of mortality decline has slowed in recent years.

All preventable deaths and injuries are tragic—those for children, especially so.

Cancer, birth defects, and influenza and pneumonia cause childhood deaths—all at relatively low rates (Figure 4-C).

No other preventable cause poses such a major threat as accidents which account for 45 percent of total childhood mortality.

By itself, a 50 percent reduction in fatal accidents would be enough to achieve the goal of fewer than 34 deaths per 100,000 by 1990. And this is not an unrealistic target, since a number of actions can be taken. It is a fact, for instance, that mandatory seat belt laws scrupulously implemented in some countries have reduced traffic accident deaths by 30 percent. It should also be entirely feasible to reduce deaths due to fires, falls, and other common childhood accidents.

In addition to disease and injury, children face other problems—of behavioral, emotional and intellectual development. They include learning difficulties, school troubles, behavioral disturbances, and speech and vision problems. A generation ago, such problems did not seem as

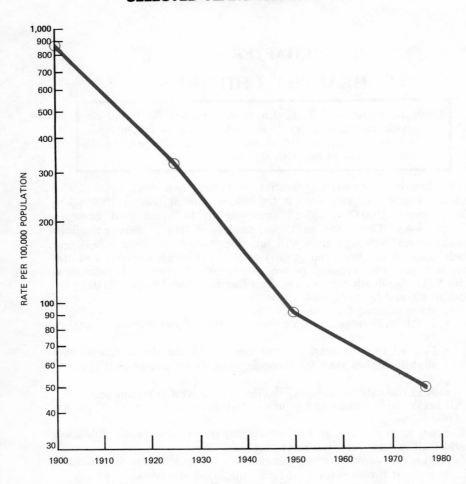

FIGURE 4-A
DEATH RATES FOR AGES 1-14 YEARS: UNITED STATES, SELECTED YEARS 1900-1977

RATE PER 100,000 POPULATION

NOTE: 1977 data are provisional; data for all other years are final. Selected years are 1900, 1925, 1950, 1977.

Source: National Center for Health Statistics, Division of Vital Statistics.

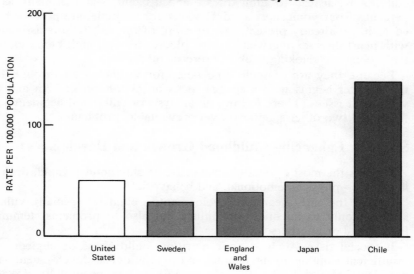

FIGURE 4-B

DEATH RATES FOR AGES 1-14 YEARS: SELECTED COUNTRIES, 1975

NOTE: The most recent year of data for Chile is 1971.

Sources: United States, National Center for Health Statistics, Division of Vital Statistics; other countries, United Nations.

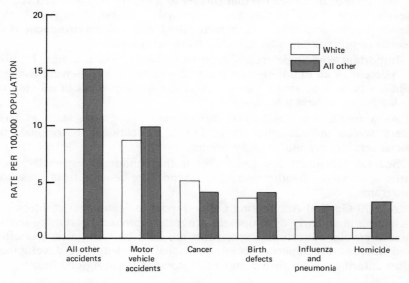

FIGURE 4-C

MAJOR CAUSES OF DEATH FOR AGES 1-14 YEARS: UNITED STATES, 1976

Source: Based on data from the National Center for Health Statistics, Division of Vital Statistics. **35**

prominent as they do today and they are now sometimes called the "new morbidity."

We must face the fact, too, that characteristics developed during childhood can lead to adult disease and disability—and as many as 40 percent of our youngsters aged 11 to 14, for example, are now estimated to have, already present, one or more of the risk factors associated with heart disease: overweight, high blood pressure, high blood cholesterol, cigarette smoking, lack of exercise, or diabetes.

Because they are of such importance for wellbeing all through life, this chapter begins with a special focus on childhood growth and development issues. There follows an analysis of childhood accidental injuries and two other significant, yet preventable, problems.

Subgoal: Enhancing Childhood Growth and Development

Perhaps the most critical characteristic of childhood is rapid, dramatic change—physical, emotional, and behavorial.

During the early years of development, a child is especially vulnerable not only to infection and injury but also to problems stemming from social or interpersonal causes.

If special risks—such as poor nutrition, child abuse or neglect, and insufficient stimulus to intellectual and psychological development—are not identified and dealt with early, growth may be profoundly affected. And the consequences of physical and psychological illness early in life, even if not apparent then, may become so later.

Is there in fact a "new morbidity?" Actually, learning disorders, inadequate school functioning, behavioral problems, and speech and vision difficulties are not new. Rather, successful control of many life-threatening childhood diseases of the past has permitted a new awareness of and sensitivity to these problems.

We have come to realize that threats to a child's physical growth and development also threaten optimal mental growth and development—and that, too, a stimulating and safe environment is essential to optimum mental growth and development.

Important sociologic trends need to be taken into account. In 1977, 18 percent of all children— up from 12 percent in 1970—were living in families headed by single parents. And almost 50 percent of all children today have mothers who work.

As a result, early childhood development programs, such as Head Start, which include an array of health, educational, nutritional, and social services are increasingly needed.

Several recent studies have shown that children, especially those from low-income families, derive many positive benefits from preschool programs.

A 1979 General Accounting Office report indicates that children participating in an early development program subsequently require less remedial special education. Participants are held back in grade less often, and demonstrate superior social, emotional and language development after entering school than comparable non-participating children.

Learning Disorders

As many as 20 percent of school age children have reading or learning disabilities which can have lifelong consequences if not overcome. They are a major cause of school dropout and can also lead to serious emotional and behavioral disturbances, some of which may be manifested as symptoms of physical illness.

Although there is little agreement on precise etiology, the consensus is that learning disabilities have multiple causes including central nervous system disorders, emotional factors, and environmental and cultural influences.

Can such disabled children be helped? Research indicates that fully 80 percent whose problems are identified early and who receive remedial education can function within normal range for their age.

Vision problems, if uncorrected, can impair learning ability—and an estimated 20 percent of all children have them. Two-thirds are nearsighted; one third, farsighted.

As much as an additional three percent have hearing difficulties, often caused by complications from middle ear infections. Impaired hearing from recurrent middle ear infections during the critical years of language development can interfere with learning ability. Early diagnosis and treatment of the infections—among the most common ailments of early childhood—could prevent many cases of temporary and some of permanent hearing damage as well as contribute to prevention of learning and behavioral problems later in childhood.

Mental Retardation

An estimated six million Americans suffer from mild to severe retardation, and each year about 100,000 children are identified as mentally retarded.

In only a small percentage of cases is retardation detectable at birth. Usually, diagnosis is made at school age. In about 90 percent of cases, the retardation is defined as mild (IQ 50 to 70).

Much mild retardation is now believed to be the result of a deprived sociocultural environment often associated with poverty; the likely mechanism: inadequate stimulation or improper nutrition. Since poor nutrition has been associated with slow mental development, it is important to ensure good nutritional habits for children.

Child Abuse and Neglect

Abuse and neglect are serious—and, unfortunately, not rare—threats to both physical and emotional development. They account not only for many injuries, burns and other seeming accidents in children but also for brain damage, emotional scars, and even deaths. There are also children who are victims of sexual abuse, incest, and rape.

The inherently intimate aspect and difficulties in identifying and reporting instances of abuse and neglect have led to widely varying estimates of their extent.

Estimates of the actual number of cases of child abuse, which is generally acknowledged to be greatly under-reported, range from 200,000 to four million a year. Child neglect is probably more common than direct physical abuse.

Abuse and neglect often appear to be manifestations of severe family instability. Stress can contribute to the instability and poverty may contribute to the stress. Alcohol is implicated in many cases. Physically or mentally handicapped children can be targets of abuse by parents frustrated by the handicaps. Parental immaturity can be critical but many otherwise stable, intelligent parents have been known to abuse their children in stressful situations.

High risk families range from the obviously deeply troubled and chronically disorganized—many already known in some way to the police or other community resources—to families temporarily under stress. Also at high risk are children of teenage mothers and those in families with closely spaced children.

Abusing parents are often immature, dependent, unable to handle responsibility. They have low self-esteem, strong beliefs about the value of physical punishment, and misconceptions about children's competence to understand and perform according to their expectations. They frequently make unreasonable demands and, during time of crisis, may direct their anger and frustration at a child. They often are isolated socially and have difficulty seeking help.

Efforts to reduce and ultimately eliminate child abuse will have to be multifaceted. Some promising approaches involve parent education, enhancement of community and social support systems, assistance to abusing parents through collaborative efforts of public and private sector, and projects designed to create an integrated health and social service delivery system. Such programs help ensure that families at risk for child abuse have continuing contact and follow-up care from a health or social services agency from the prenatal period through the school years.

Nutrition

The nutritional habits developed in childhood can profoundly affect health throughout life.

No longer are overt nutritional deficiencies as common as they once were, particularly among the poor and uneducated, although iron deficiency still exists among disadvantaged children and may show up during screening examinations. To some extent, the needs of children who would otherwise be undernourished have been met by school programs which provide nutritious breakfasts and lunches, and by food stamps or income supplements. Improvements in these programs, however, are required to more adequately meet needs.

Today's most prevalent nutritional problems are overeating and ill-advised food choices. Obesity—a risk factor for hypertension, heart disease and diabetes—frequently begins during childhood. About one-third of today's obese adults were overweight as children. An obese child is at least three times more likely than another to be an obese adult. Because obesity is more difficult to correct in adulthood, major preventive efforts are best directed toward children and adolescents.

Another cause of concern is the diet of a large proportion of today's children—containing considerably more fat and sugar than a reasonable diet should have. Underscoring the seriousness of that concern is evidence of coronary arteriosclerosis in seemingly healthy young people in their late teens. Limiting fat consumption by children may reduce blood fat levels and, thus, a risk factor for heart disease.

Subgoal: Reducing Childhood Accidents and Injuries

Almost 10,000 American children aged one to 14 were killed in accidents in 1977, more than three times as many as died from the next leading cause of death, cancer.

Motor vehicle accidents are responsible for more than 20 percent of childhood deaths, drownings for eight percent, and fires for six percent.

Although these problems fall under the rubric of health, they are the results primarily of environmental and social factors—and thus not amenable to usual medical intervention.

Prevention requires changes in the behavioral patterns of many parents as well as children. Frequently, accidents result from the poor judgment of parents who, for example, speed or drive after drinking—and from failure to teach proper precautionary measures to children.

But attention to other factors, such as motor vehicle and highway design, can reduce motor vehicle accident risk—and safety measures can cut the toll of accidental deaths from drownings and fires.

Most accidents among older children are accounted for by recreational activities and equipment. Among leading causes of the 498,000 recorded emergency room visits made by children aged six to 11 in 1976, were bicycle, swing, and skateboard accidents. For those 12 to 17, the leading causes included football, basketball, and bicycle riding. Contact sport injuries, it should be noted, often involve the mouth and teeth—and the aftereffects and treatment may be long and costly.

Toxic substances in the home—drugs, cleaning agents, pesticides, and other items—pose a special hazard to younger children. Although childhood poisoning deaths have been reduced in the past decade through changes in the formulation and packaging of poisonous agents, poisoning still accounts for five percent of non-motor vehicle accidental deaths among children under five.

Lead poisoning is a particularly striking example of an environmental hazard with severe consequences for children. Each year, ingestion or inhalation of lead leads to central nervous system damage or mental retardation in 6,000 children as well as death for another 300 to 400.

Although it is a potential hazard for all children, lead poisoning is especially threatening for inner city children who may be more vulnerable because of lead ingested in paint chips from peeling, dilapidated walls as well as lead inhaled from automobile exhausts. Elevated lead levels have been detected in the blood and teeth of as many as 25 percent of children aged one to six living in neighborhoods with deteriorating housing. Research has been revealing an association between high blood or body lead levels and learning disabilities.

Other Important Problems

Still prominent threats to the good health of children include two other areas susceptible to preventive interventions: vaccine-preventable diseases and dental health.

Vaccine-Preventable Diseases

We have come tantalizingly close but have yet to reach a feasible goal: to protect all American children from the many serious diseases and the permanent physical and mental handicaps they may cause for which effective immunization is available.

That the goal of virtually eliminating such diseases is feasible and that intensive systematic immunization can achieve it is perhaps most dramatically demonstrated by the worldwide elimination of smallpox. Another prominent example: the decline in paralytic polio, since vaccine introduction in 1955, from as many as 20,000 cases a year in the 1940s and early 1950s to seven cases in 1978.

Today, measles is considered the most threatening of the childhood contagious diseases which remain both prevalent and preventable. Its frequent complications include pneumonia, ear infections and deafness. Brain inflammation (encephalitis) occurs in about one of every 1,000 cases, often producing permanent brain damage and mental retardation. About one of every 10,000 children afflicted with measles dies as a result of complications.

In 1962, there were nearly five million cases of measles (of which about 500,000 were officially reported). After the introduction of the measles vaccine in 1963, reported measles incidence was reduced by more than 90 percent.

In recent years the number of cases reported has ranged from 22,000 in 1974 to 57,000 in 1977. But, as a result of the recent National Childhood Immunization Initiative, the incidence of measles has experienced a remarkable decline to the lowest levels ever recorded.

Rubella (German measles) remains a problem of importance, with 20,000 reported cases in 1977 (actual cases are estimated to be as much as 20 times the reported number). The most dangerous consequence of rubella is damage to the fetus when a woman becomes infected early in pregnancy (see Chapter 3). A vaccine is available and immunization of children—and of young women before pregnancy—is vital.

Mumps, although usually not a serious disease in childhood, nevertheless can sometimes involve the central nervous system, with nerve deafness as one of the most severe complications. Approximately one case of deafness occurs for every 15,000 cases of mumps in the United States. In adults, mumps can affect the reproductive organs and in males this occasionally results in sterility. A combined vaccine—for mumps, measles and rubella—makes immunization against mumps practical. Still, more than 16,000 cases occurred in 1978.

For diphtheria, pertussis (whooping cough) and tetanus (lockjaw), vaccines are readily available. Yet, while incidence has dropped to low levels, many children remain unprotected and vulnerable to the respiratory, cardiovascular, and nervous system complications which may occur with these diseases.

Pertussis was a leading cause of death for children at the turn of the century. Today it is fatal to one of every 100 children reported afflicted, but only 2,000 cases were reported in 1977. Diphtheria and tetanus occur less frequently (under 100 reported cases of each in 1977). Still, all three diseases remain threats for children not adequately immunized.

Prior to the national childhood immunization effort which began in 1977, one-quarter to one-half of pre-school and school-age children remained incompletely immunized. Ironically, the great success of previous immunization programs created a complacency and was one reason why many children were not being immunized. The gains of the past two years demonstrated that national and local campaigns are needed on a sustained basis to increase parental awareness of the need for immunization and maintain immunization at an acceptable level.

Contagious diseases for which immunizations are available are not the only childhood infectious diseases of concern. Rheumatic fever—caused by streptococcal infection—ranked 40 years ago as the leading cause of death for children aged five to 15. Today, with early diagnosis and adequate treatment for streptococcal infections, complications such as rheumatic fever can be prevented.

Dental Health

Tooth decay affects most children soon after age three when the primary teeth have appeared. By age 11, the average American child has three permanent teeth damaged by decay. By age 17, eight or nine permanent teeth have decayed, been filled, or are missing.

Tooth decay is irreversible. Once begun, decay that is left untreated usually destroys the tooth. Although treatment generally consists of removing the decay and filling the tooth, the problem is compounded by frequent recurrence within relatively brief periods of time. Follow-up and continuing detection and treatment are needed.

Even though decay primarily occurs in childhood, it may lead to misalignment or loss later of permanent teeth. It can also affect appearance and lead to nutrition and speech problems, and difficulties in normal emotional development.

Decay has three requisites: a susceptible tooth, a population of certain bacteria in the mouth, and certain foods, particularly sugars, to encourage the bacteria. Prevention efforts, therefore, must be aimed at making teeth less susceptible, minimizing bacterial growth, and altering the diet.

The biggest problems are sweets, particularly sticky sweets and hard candies. Sugary materials that are eaten frequently, or that remain in the mouth for extended periods, encourage bacteria in the mouth to form acids that destroy tooth enamel, and subsequently, underlying tooth structures. The practice of giving an infant or small child a bedtime bottle filled with milk or sweet liquid also is conducive to decay.

That reduction of sugar intake can avoid much decay was demonstrated by the significant decline in tooth decay in European countries during the two World Wars when sugar was in short supply.

Many children also experience disease of the supporting tissues (periodontal disease). Usually beginning in childhood, periodontal disease progresses slowly and, unless checked, can cause serious problems later in life, including complete loss of teeth.

Fluoridation has demonstrated over the past 30 years that it is one of the most effective measures in preventing tooth decay and is addressed in Chapter 9.

• • • •

Many factors affect a child's development— genetics, the home environment, the quality of interactions with parents, teachers, health professionals, other adults, peers. With so many influences, no single course of action will protect the future mental, emotional, and physical health of every child and assure realization of full developmental potential. Section III will detail needed actions.

But the special importance of the school should be emphasized here.

Many hours of a child's life are spent in the classroom. Providing health services through school programs can be of great value; so could effective health education.

Our children could benefit greatly from a basic understanding of the human body and its functioning, needs, and potential—and from an understanding of what really is involved in health and disease.

There are a number of school systems which have developed good models for health education.

For other schools to really take on what could be their highly significant role in health education and health promotion will require a commitment by school leadership at local, State and national levels to apply these models.

CHAPTER 5

HEALTHY ADOLESCENTS AND YOUNG ADULTS

> **Goal:** To improve the health and health habits of adolescents and young adults, and, by 1990, to reduce deaths among people ages 15 to 24 by at least 20 percent, to fewer than 93 per 100,000.

Obviously enough, adolescence is a period of complex changes—in physical growth and maturation and in transition from childhood dependency to adult autonomy.

In health, it is—relatively—a good period as measured by the usual morbidity and mortality indicators. Although the death rate for the 40 million young Americans in the 15 to 24 year age group is 2.5 times the rate for children, it is substantially below that for other age groups.

Yet, while health for this age group, as for others, is considerably better than 75 years ago (Figure 5-A), there is one startling difference: for adolescents and young adults, recent progress has not been sustained, as it has been for other age groups.

Americans aged 15 to 24 now have a higher death rate than 20 years ago.

In 1960, the adolescent/young adult mortality rate was 106 deaths per 100,000. By 1970, the rate was up to 128. By 1976, it had dropped to 113—but 1977 statistics show an increase again to 117. This represents nearly 48,000 deaths in 1977 alone. Americans aged 15 to 24 have a higher death rate than their counterparts in other countries such as Sweden, England and Wales, and Japan (Figure 5-B).

What are the principal threats to health? Violent death and injury, alcohol and drug abuse, unwanted pregnancies, sexually transmissible diseases are among the more common health-related problems for this age group.

Young men are at particular risk, their death rate being almost three times that of young women. And, although chronic diseases are not among the major causes of death at this period of life (Figure 5-C), the lifestyles and behavior patterns which are shaped during these years may determine later susceptibility to chronic diseases.

Accidents, homicides, and suicides account for about three-fourths of all deaths in this age group. Responsibility has been attributed to behavior patterns characterized by judgmental errors, aggressiveness, and, in some cases, ambivalence about wanting to live or die. Certainly, greater risk-taking occurs in this period of life.

FIGURE 5-A

DEATH RATES FOR AGES 15-24 YEARS: UNITED STATES, SELECTED YEARS 1900-1977

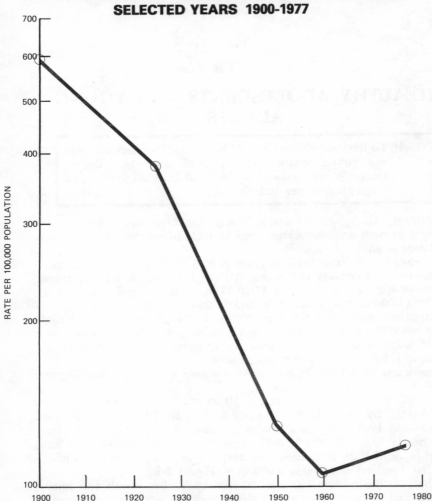

NOTE: 1977 data are provisional; data for all other years are final. Selected years are 1900, 1925, 1950, 1960, 1977.

Source: National Center for Health Statistics, Division of Vital Statistics.

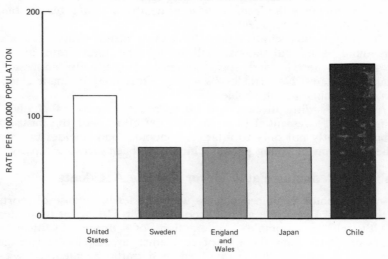

FIGURE 5-B
DEATH RATES FOR AGES 15-24 YEARS:
SELECTED COUNTRIES, 1975

NOTE: The most recent year of data for Chile is 1971.

Sources: United States, National Center for Health Statistics, Division of Vital Statistics; other countries, United Nations.

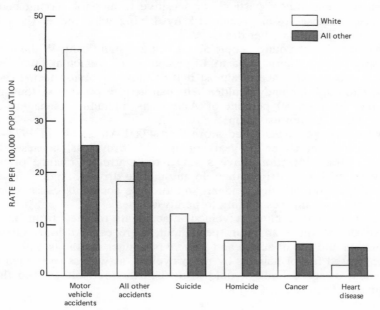

FIGURE 5-C
MAJOR CAUSES OF DEATH FOR AGES 15-24 YEARS:
UNITED STATES, 1976

Source: Based on data from the National Center for Health Statistics, Division of Vital Statistics.

The variability of these traumatic deaths by sex and race is striking. All types are three to four times more frequent for males. While motor vehicle accident deaths are more likely to occur among white youths, young blacks of either sex are at least five times as likely to be murdered; homicide is the leading cause of death for young blacks, ranking slightly ahead of total accidents.

Certainly, injury control must be a clear health promotion priority for young people but the task will not be easy. Injury rates are linked to factors—lifestyle and socioeconomic—not usually addressed by health programs. Nevertheless, a strong effort must be made since this is a major public health problem.

An equally difficult task will be to reduce misuse of alcohol and drugs. But it is essential to strengthen the effort—for the misuse contributes greatly not only to injuries, homicides and suicides but also to other problems of young people which have been growing rapidly.

Subgoal: Reducing Fatal Motor Vehicle Accidents

In 1977 motor vehicle accidents were the leading cause of mortality in the 15 to 24 year age group, accounting for 37 percent of all deaths.

Although a complex interaction—of driver, vehicle and roadway—determines the risk of accidents, nevertheless a teenage or young adult driver who is involved in a traffic accident is twice as likely to die as a driver 25 years old or older.

Alcohol consumption is clearly implicated in many of the fatalities. About half of fatally injured drivers have been found to have blood alcohol concentrations of more than 100 mg/dl (100 milligrams of alcohol per deciliter of blood). In most states, this is considered presumptive evidence of intoxication. Blood alcohol levels even lower than 100 mg/dl increase the likelihood of an accident— especially for teenagers, the elderly, and others particularly sensitive to alcohol. Young people also place themselves at greater risk by driving while under the influence of marijuana or other drugs.

The attitudes of young people about risk are significant. While excessive speed was a factor in 35 to 40 percent of all vehicular fatalities in 1977, it was an influence in almost half of those involving teenagers 15 to 19. Although lap and shoulder belts can help to prevent serious injuries and fatalities, 80 percent of Americans, including teenagers and young adults, do not use them.

Motorcycle accidents killed more than 4,000 Americans in 1977—30 percent of them under 20 years of age. Motorcyclists, because they have so little protection, have a seven times greater chance of fatal injury for each mile driven than do automobile drivers. And, more frequently than automobile accidents, motorcycle accidents cause severe, permanent head injuries leading to paralysis.

Although some decline in vehicular accidents resulted from institution of the 55 miles an hour speed limit, more can be done. Greater production and use of active and passive passenger restraints, safer cars, and increased use of helmets by motorcyclists, as well as continued enforcement of speed limits, would lead to further reductions, and these actions are discussed in Chapter 9.

Subgoal: Reducing Alcohol and Drug Misuse

Alcohol and drug abuse are behaviors with major implications in many areas. Not only do they increase risk of accidents, suicides, and homicides, they also contribute to family disruption and poor school and job performance; and they have a potential for leading to long-term chronic disease.

Use of alcohol and drugs has been increasing among young people. About 80 percent of 12 to 17 year olds report having had a drink, more than half drink at least once a month, nearly three percent drink daily. Since 1966, the number of high school students intoxicated at least once a month has more than doubled, from 10 to over 20 percent. Nearly 80 percent of male high school seniors drink at least once a month and more than six percent drink daily.

Although young people may drink less regularly than older people, they tend to consume larger quantities and are more likely to become intoxicated on drinking occasions. No wonder, then, that alcohol-related accidents are the leading cause of death in the 15 to 24 age group and 60 percent of all alcohol-related highway traffic fatalities are among young people.

Drug abuse was virtually unknown among young people in 1950. Prior to 1962, lifetime experience with any illicit drug was limited to less than two percent of the population, including young people.

By 1977, 60 percent of 18 to 25 year olds had tried marijuana; about 20 percent had tried stronger substances such as cocaine and hallucinogens; and about 30 percent had illegally used drugs available only on medical prescription. Even among 12 to 17 year olds, nearly 30 percent had tried marijuana.

Beyond increasing drug experimentation among young people, the frequency of use is increasing. Less than one percent of high school students report daily use of drugs other than alcohol, tobacco or marijuana—but over 20 percent regularly smoke cigarettes and about 10 percent smoke marijuana every day. And stimulants—amphetamines—are another category of drugs which young people report taking most frequently.

The physical and psychological effects are highly variable. They differ from person to person as well as from drug to drug. It is, therefore difficult to determine precisely how harmful experimentation is in terms of the drug use to which it leads.

By any measure, however, drug problems are serious, have increased greatly—and if the full potential of our adolescents and young adults is to be realized, additional steps (Chapter 10) must be taken to reduce the harmful effects from both alcohol and drugs.

Other Important Problems

Among other prominent threats to the physical and mental health of young people are problems of adolescent pregnancy, sexually transmissible diseases, mental illness, suicide and homicide. To a great extent, they represent failures to help young people acquire the skills and information needed to solve problems and make sound decisions during years of rapid change.

Teenage Pregnancy

Childbearing during adolescence is a high risk experience for mother and child alike.

Yet one-fourth of American teenage girls have had at least one pregnancy by age 19. Every year about one million adolescents under the age of 19 become pregnant, including perhaps 300,000 under 15—which represents an annual rate of 10 percent of all teenage girls. Two-thirds of them are unmarried. At least three of every 10 elect to terminate their pregnancies. Birth rates for teenagers aged 16 to 19 are declining but they are increasing for girls under 16.

These young mothers have greater risk of bearing low birth weight infants—with consequent developmental problems and risk of infant death associated with low birth weight, as noted in Chapter 3. And often they face significant social problems: disruption of schooling, high rates of repeat pregnancy, and public dependency.

A substantial proportion of school districts still encourage expectant teenage mothers to drop out of school; many do not provide for continuing education; more than 25 percent of the young mothers become pregnant again within just a year after their first delivery.

A major underlying problem that urgently needs addressing for this age group is the inadequate knowledge of, and access to, information on sexual behavior and family planning services. In 1976, an estimated 40 percent of unmarried teenage girls, aged 15 to 19 (two-thirds by age 19), had engaged in sexual intercourse and 25 percent of them never used any form of contraception.

Birth control methods currently prevent an estimated 750,000 unwanted pregnancies annually. If all sexually active young people who do not want to become pregnant were to use some effective form of contraception regularly, it is estimated that premarital pregnancies would drop by more than 300,000 a year.

There is growing evidence, too, that for the pregnant teenager and her baby, comprehensive programs, which include emphasis on the mother's continued schooling, are associated with fewer repeat pregnancies. Many programs have been developed which demonstrate the value of education for parenthood and family planning—and of improved family support for teenage parents.

An example of what a medical center-based program for teen mothers and their infants can accomplish is provided by a program at the Johns Hopkins Medical Institutions in Baltimore.

There, staff members provide young mothers with comprehensive medical and psychological services, conduct classes from the first prenatal visit through labor, delivery, and for three years after delivery, and, perhaps most important, form close supportive relationships with the young women.

Recent results indicate that 85 percent of mothers enrolled at the center have returned to school and only five percent became pregnant again within a year after delivery. Of all Baltimore teen mothers, only

10 percent return to school and 47 percent become pregnant again within a year. Teen mothers in the program also have had fewer obstetrical complications and fewer premature deliveries, and have given birth to larger and healthier babies than Baltimore's teen mothers in general.

Sexually Transmissible Diseases

Sexually transmissible diseases increasingly threaten the health and well-being of millions of adolescents and young adults.

Although there has been some recent improvement, overall, in the incidence of gonorrhea and syphilis, both diseases continue to increase among adolescents.

Moreover, other sexually transmissible diseases—such as genital herpes and nonspecific urethritis—have recently become recognized as major public health problems. Along with gonorrhea and syphilis, they account for an estimated eight to 12 million cases of sexually transmitted diseases a year.

And the greatest risk of acquiring them occurs among young people age 15 to 24 who account for about 75 percent of all cases.

Because infection is often unrecognized for lack of apparent symptoms, many young people also suffer serious permanent complications. Each year, an estimated 75,000 women of childbearing age become sterile as a result of pelvic inflammatory disease caused by a sexually transmitted infection. Actions to control sexually transmissible diseases are discussed in Chapter 8.

Mental Health

That adolescents today are coming of age in a predominantly urban, technological society, characterized in part by shifting values and traditions, may account in no small part for alcohol and drug abuse problems and others.

Since individual development does not take place in a vacuum but is strongly influenced by sociocultural factors, society's expectations play a large part in the way young people experience this period of their lives. But the turbulence of the last decade has made it difficult for young people to develop any clear sense of what these expectations are.

Some observers point to teenage pregnancy, delinquency and crime, suicides, and child abuse as well as drug and alcohol abuse as both evidence and products of that uncertainty. Others contend that these problems are simply more visible today and involve only a minority of adolescents.

In any event, the transition from childhood to adulthood may take some toll on an adolescent's emotional stability. And problems such as 20 percent unemployment among teenagers (40 percent for minority youth) create additional stress for young people trying to develop their identity and their place in life.

While the full degree of impact of broad social issues and overall social and national stability on personal development is not clear, there is general agreement that the family has the most direct influence on the expectations of young people. Yet family structures have been undergoing significant changes in recent years.

Added complexity is faced by the teenage parent, often single, trying to fulfill the personal growth needs of an adolescent while simultaneously having to meet the needs of a dependent, rapidly developing baby. Because of the demands of these responsibilities, support through special programs for teenage parents, including some form of day care and other community and mental health services, is very much needed.

The diverse problems of teenagers and young adults require a broad range of mental health services and the combined efforts of the family, school, workplace, and community. The pressures of parents and peers, as well as of the media, are all factors which contribute to these problems—and which can be employed to help solve them.

The growth of community mental health services in recent decades has made resources more available in local areas and adolescents are gradually beginning to use them. But mental health programs tailored to adolescents are not abundantly available. The recent report of the President's Commission on Mental Health recommends expansion of these programs.

Suicide

Suicide is the third leading cause of death among teenagers and young adults, some 5,600 of whom took their own lives in 1977. Of total suicides, 20 percent are committed by people under age 25.

Among adults, three times as many men as women commit suicide and adolescent males are more likely to take their own lives than adolescent females.

The most frequent weapons include firearms, drugs, and motor vehicle exhaust gases. Firearms are used four times as often as poisoning (the second most frequent method), and firearm suicides have been increasing at a much faster rate than suicides by other means.

Unfortunately the suicide rate among young people has not plateaued, but is increasing. In 1950, the rate was only about 20 percent of what it reached in 1977. In 1976, more than one of every 10 teenagers and young adults who died committed suicide. Many more suicides were attempted but not reported as such or not identified as suicidal efforts.

It is estimated that some five million Americans have made one or more unsuccessful attempts at suicide and that 10 percent of this group will ultimately succeed. Some estimates indicate that the actual suicide rate is three times the reported rate.

An increased suicide rate is not unique to this country. Many other industrialized nations are experiencing increases, particularly among young people. Indeed, in 1974 several countries exceeded the United States suicide rate of about 12 deaths per 100,000. Japan had 18, Sweden 20, and Germany 21.

Most suicidal persons give verbal or behavioral warnings first, and 80 percent of those who take their own lives have made previous attempts. While predicting suicide with certainty is impossible, those at highest risk include people who are severely depressed and those at odds with themselves and the people close to them. Mental health workers are becoming more skillful in early detection and management of suicidal tendencies. A prime need is for hotlines—and prompt referral to sources of professional help when problems are noted (see Chapter 10).

Homicide

Murder accounts for over 10 percent of all deaths among adolescents and young adults—just under seven percent for whites but almost 30 percent for blacks in this age group.

In 1977, when an estimated 21,000 Americans were victims of homicide, about 25 percent were aged 15 to 24, placing that group at greater risk than the rest of the population. The deaths of these young people represent a very large and tragic waste in terms of the many years of productive life lost with each death.

The American homicide rate is very much greater than for most other industrialized nations. Our rate of 10.2 homicides per 100,000 people in 1974 compares with a rate of only 0.9 for France, 1.0 for Great Britain, 1.1 for Sweden, and 1.3 for Japan.

In about 20 percent of murders in this country, victim and offender are relatives or have a close relationship; in 40 percent, they are acquaintances; and in the remaining 40 percent, there is no known relationship. An estimated 60 to 80 percent of homicides occur as the result of personal disagreements and conflict, while robbery, sexual assault and other circumstances account for the rest.

As with other fatal injuries, homicide is more common among the poor, more frequent on weekends and at night, and often associated with alcohol abuse. In about 90 percent of murders, both offender and victim are of the same race. Men are three to four times more likely to be victims—and five times as likely to be offenders—as women.

Many factors undoubtedly are involved in our high homicide rate. Economic deprivation, family breakup, the glamorizing of violence in the media, and the availability of handguns all are important. Firearms, the most frequently used homicide weapon in the United States, were involved in 63 percent of the murders occurring in 1977, with handguns used in half, and cutting or stabbing weapons employed in 18 percent.

Easy access to firearms appears to be the one factor with a striking relationship to murder. From 1960 to 1974, handgun sales quadrupled to more than six million a year. During that same period, the homicide rate increased from 4.7 per 100,000 to 10.2 for the overall population—and from 5.9 to 14.2 for young people aged 15 to 24.

• • • •

Broad physical, psychological, social, and family changes all have a powerful impact on young people.

Young people are compelled to adjust not only to rapid individual changes, but simultaneously to meet the expectations of both family and community. The strains which result can have considerable bearing on the problems of adolescents and young adults.

Stress is to be expected in life. But for some adolescents and young adults, it can become overwhelming.

At critical junctures, they urgently need assistance in finding ways to cope and make important decisions and constructive adjustments. Such assistance (described in Chapter 10) can contribute greatly to improving both their health and the quality and value of their lives.

CHAPTER 6

HEALTHY ADULTS

Goal: To improve the health of adults, and, by 1990, to reduce deaths among people ages 25 to 64 by at least 25 percent, to fewer than 400 per 100,000.

The contrast is sharp. For an infant at birth, life expectancy since 1900 has increased 26 years. But today for a man at age 45 the expectancy is only five years greater than it was in 1900.

On the one hand, preventive measures have been successful in reducing infant and childhood deaths from what were the major threats in those years, the acute contagious diseases. On the other hand, treatment measures, even though increasingly sophisticated, have been far less successful against what are the prime threats for adults: the chronic diseases, often of insidious onset, slowly progressive, ultimately devastating.

Only recently have we gained significant insights into the causes and many risk factors involved in the chronic diseases—and into tangible, applicable preventive measures. Although those measures are different and the results may be less immediately dramatic than was the case for the acute childhood diseases, we already have reason for optimism in what has been happening very recently to adult mortality trends.

In 1970, the death rate for adults aged 25 to 64 was even higher than in 1960—657 per 100,000, up from 640.

Since then, however, there has been an annual average decrease of 2.6 percent in the death rate for adults. By 1976, the rate had dropped to 555. And data for 1977 show a further 2.7 percent decrease to 540 (Figure 6-A).

More than one-third of all deaths among the 100 million American adults have been due to cardiovascular diseases, principally coronary artery (heart) disease and stroke (Figure 6-C). And it is deaths from those causes which have been declining and accounting for most of the drop in mortality rate.

There is every reason to believe that the downward trend not only can be maintained but accelerated with increased efforts on behalf of such preventive measures as high blood pressure detection and control, reduction of smoking, prudent diet, increased exercise and fitness, and better stress management.

A reduction in cancer deaths should also be achievable—to a worthwhile, even if necessarily more limited, extent in the near future.

FIGURE 6-A

DEATH RATES FOR AGES 25-64 YEARS: UNITED STATES, SELECTED YEARS 1900-1977

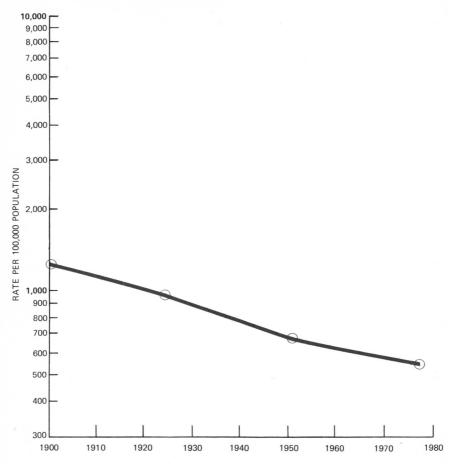

NOTE: 1977 data are provisional; data for all other years are final. Selected years are 1900, 1925, 1950, 1977.

Source: National Center for Health Statistics, Division of Vital Statistics.

54

FIGURE 6-B

DEATH RATES FOR AGES 25-64 YEARS: SELECTED COUNTRIES, 1975

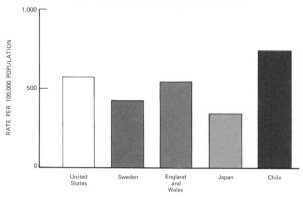

NOTE: The most recent year of data for Chile is 1971.

Sources: United States, National Center for Health Statistics, Division of Vital Statistics; other countries, United Nations.

FIGURE 6-C

MAJOR CAUSES OF DEATH FOR AGES 25-64 YEARS: UNITED STATES, 1976

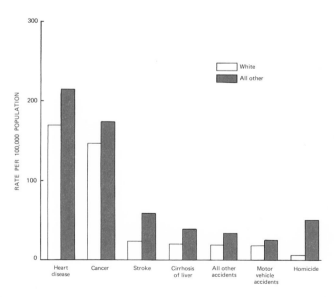

Source: Based on data from the National Center for Health Statistics, Division of Vital Statistics.

One reason for slower progress against cancer is that by the time malignancy becomes apparent, many years have gone into its development. In a sense, any currently appearing cancer reflects past history—perhaps, for example, 35 years of smoking in a 55-year-old patient with lung cancer. Therefore, it will take years for modifications of cancer risk factors to be expressed in marked reductions in cancer mortality.

A second reason is that declining rates for certain cancers will be more than offset by increases in occupational and smoking-related malignancies because of already-established adverse effects. The net result will be a small, gradual rise for the next few years in the age-adjusted death rate for cancer.

Prevention efforts—to reduce exposure to cancer-inducing agents and to foster more early detection and prompt treatment—need to be instituted now to reverse the trend.

Subgoal: Reducing Heart Attacks and Strokes

In 1977, heart disease was responsible for over 700,000 deaths—the leading cause of death for men after age 40. And although women, up to menopause, have about one-third the heart disease rate of men, their heart attack incidence thereafter increases, begins to approach the male rate by age 70, and virtually equals it by age 85.

Heart disease not only produces fatal heart attacks; it is also the greatest cause of permanent disability claims among workers under 65, and responsible for more days of hospitalization than any other single disorder. And it is the principal cause of limited activity for some 2.5 million Americans under age 65.

Stroke, in 1977, led to nearly 183,000 deaths, almost 10 percent of the total mortality for the year. Although some 250,000 Americans survive strokes each year, many remain disabled by paralysis, speech difficulties, and memory loss. Nearly 10 percent of nursing home admissions in people under 65 are because of strokes.

Although most stroke deaths (about 85 percent) occur in people over 65, early deaths are not uncommon, particularly among blacks who, between ages 25 and 64, have a stroke death rate almost 2.5 times that of whites.

But we are now beginning to see a welcome decline in death rates for both heart disease and strokes.

For heart disease, the death rate, which had been increasing rapidly after 1940 began to level off in the early 1960s and, between 1968 and 1977, fell by 22 percent. For stroke, the death rate, declining gradually over the last two decades, dipped more sharply, falling off 32 percent, between 1968 and 1977.

Behind both diseases lies the process of atherosclerosis in which critical arteries become narrowed by fatty deposits. Beginning silently, even as early as the first decade of life, atherosclerosis gradually thickens the walls of affected arteries with "plaques" which usually consist of a core of cholesterol and fats. The wall thickening progressively narrows artery diameter, reducing the amount of oxygen-carrying blood reaching the heart, brain or other parts of the body.

56

Manifestations do not usually appear until the disease process is well advanced and blood flow considerably reduced. Chest pain (angina pectoris) may appear when excitement, physical effort, or exposure to cold increases the heart's requirements for oxygen beyond the level that can be supplied by the impaired blood flow. Angina may be a forerunner of eventual heart attack—but heart attacks, frequently fatal, can occur suddenly, without warning, when an already narrowed coronary artery serving the heart is further blocked, completely shutting off flow to an area of the heart muscle.

A stroke occurs when the blood and oxygen supply to the brain is severely reduced. The mechanism can be similar to that of a heart attack—further blocking of an artery supplying brain tissue, usually an artery already compromised by atherosclerosis. Most strokes are of this type. A stroke may also occur when an artery ruptures in the brain and the hemorrhaging destroys brain tissue.

Risk Factors for Heart Disease and Stroke

The importance of risk factors is not in question. Each individually is clearly linked to increased likelihood of heart disease or stroke—and in combination they multiply the likelihood. What only remains uncertain is the precise extent to which risk can be decreased by modifying the risk factors.

Smoking. Since the late 1940s, research has consistently shown that cigarette smokers have nearly twice the heart disease death rate of non-smokers. The difference is much greater in individuals under 65.

Substances in cigarette smoke which may be hazardous to the heart include nicotine and carbon monoxide.

Risk is proportional to the amount of smoke inhaled and the number of cigarettes smoked. Smokers of more than one pack a day are three times more likely to experience a heart attack than non-smokers (Figure 6-D). Pipe and cigar smokers have only slightly higher rates of coronary heart disease than non-smokers.

Hypertension. High blood pressure contributes to heart disease by putting an added burden on the heart which must pump against the increased pressure in the arteries and it also seems to be a factor in the thickening of artery walls. Hypertension increases risk of stroke by promoting the atherosclerotic process in arteries supplying the brain—and by contributing to the rupture of relatively fragile brain vessels.

A blood pressure measurement consistently over 140 systolic (the pressure when the heart contracts) and 90 diastolic (the pressure when the heart relaxes between beats) is usually considered abnormal. And people with pressures exceeding 160/95 are considered to have hypertension which would benefit from treatment. About 35 million Americans have pressures above 160/95.

A study in Framingham, Massachusetts, has shown that men aged 45 to 64 who have pressures of above 160/95 have two to three times the coronary heart disease rate of those with pressures under 140/90. Among people with systolic pressures above 160, strokes are three times as frequent as among those with systolic pressures under 140.

FIGURE 6D

AGE-ADJUSTED RATES OF FIRST HEART ATTACK
BY SMOKING STATUS FOR WHITE MALES
AGES 30-59 YEARS: UNITED STATES

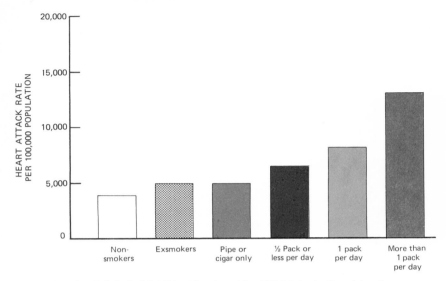

NOTE: Age-adjusted to the United States white male population, 1960. Data based on the pooled results
of five longitudinal investigations conducted in the 1950's and 1960's. Rates based on ten-year followup.

Source: National Cooperative Pooling Project, National Heart, Lung, and Blood Institute, 1970.

The high incidence of stroke deaths at younger ages among blacks is probably due in large measure to the increased prevalence and severity of hypertension which occurs in black Americans for reasons not yet clear.

Cholesterol. Premature heart disease is unequivocally associated with elevated blood cholesterol levels. Stroke risk, too, is increased by elevated serum cholesterol, although the association is not as strong as for heart disease.

For American men, the average cholesterol level is about 220 mg/dl (milligrams of cholesterol in a deciliter of blood). Heart attacks are five times as frequent in men—and women—aged 35 to 44 who have cholesterol levels above 265 as among those with levels below 220. In general, the lower one's blood cholesterol the less the likelihood of heart disease; the higher the cholesterol level, the greater the risk.

It is cholesterol deposited from the blood which goes into atherosclerotic plaques. And cholesterol carrier substances in the blood, called lipoproteins, have recently been found to play an important role in atherosclerotic disease. One type—low-density lipoproteins (LDL)—appears to accelerate cholesterol deposition in artery walls. However, another type—high-density lipoproteins (HDL)—appears not to hasten the process, and may even be protective.

58

Current research suggests that measuring HDL and LDL levels may be a more accurate means of predicting risk for atherosclerosis and heart attack than measuring serum cholesterol alone. Factors like exercise and perhaps even simple dietary modifications may increase the ratio of HDL to LDL and thereby possibly protect against heart disease.

Direct evidence from animal studies supports the linkage of atherosclerosis with high levels of fats (particularly saturated) and cholesterol in the diet.

Diabetes. Diabetes is a fourth important risk factor for cardiovascular disease. Diabetics have more severe atherosclerosis, twice as many heart attacks, and about twice as many strokes as nondiabetics of the same age. For diabetic women, the risk of atherosclerotic disease is five times greater than for other women.

Diabetics are also more likely to be hypertensive and overweight. Control of blood pressure and elimination of smoking are especially important for them since these risk factors still further heighten their premature death rate.

Other risk factors. Although they may be somewhat less important in their effects than the four major risk factors just noted, other risk factors for coronary heart disease include overweight, physical inactivity, personality patterns which are related to stress, genetic predisposition, and oral contraceptive use.

Even a moderate excess of weight may be associated with increased levels of very low-density lipoproteins in the blood and with high blood pressure and high blood sugar. Still undetermined is whether physical inactivity—which may be associated with excess weight and elevated blood cholesterol, sugar, and blood pressure levels— independently increases the risk of premature heart attack or stroke.

All people face ordinary stresses of life and work. Some, however, invoke additional, extraordinary stresses. Typically, they are extremely ambitious, competitive, and impatient, and some studies indicate that they are at higher risk of coronary heart disease.

In some families, early heart attacks—before age 50—affect several closely related members, leading to the belief that a genetic predisposition to heart disease may exist. Hypertension, diabetes, and serum cholesterol abnormalities are, in some cases, known to be hereditary, but other genetic factors adding to heart disease risk have yet to be identified. Children of parents who have had heart attacks before age 50 can be tested for relatively rare hereditary fat metabolism disorders. For most people, however, any contribution to risk made by genetic conditions is exacerbated by cigarette smoking, poor dietary habits, and other behavior that members of a family often share in common.

Some drugs may increase risk. A substantial increase has been noted in women who use oral contraceptives or estrogen replacements, and who may have other risk associations. For example, women aged 40 to 44 who both use oral contraceptives and smoke have about 10 times the risk of death from heart attack as women who do neither.

Subgoal: Reducing Death from Cancer

Cancer, the disease most feared by Americans and developed by one in four, claimed nearly 390,000 lives in 1977, making it the second most common cause of death. More than a third of deaths occur in the middle years (ages 35 to 64) of life. Although far more frequent among adults, cancer also occurs in children.

The most common fatal cancers are: leukemia, kidney and nervous system malignancies in children; lung, intestine and breast cancer in adults; and cancer of the intestine, lung, prostate and uterus in older Americans. Almost half of all cancer fatalities in the United States are from three varieties: lung, large intestine, and breast.

All cancers are similar in apparently occurring when body cells begin to multiply without the usual internal restraints. The malignant cells push the normal out of the way, spread out, and even migrate to distant parts of the body.

The process can be relatively quick, as in some forms of leukemia. But for the most common types, including breast cancer, it is believed that 10, 15, even 25 years may pass before all of the steps in the biological chain of events leading to cancer are completed. Once they are, varying lengths of time may elapse before enough cancerous cells accumulate to be recognized.

Cancer is not a single disease but rather a group of diseases occurring worldwide in man and all other mammalian species. Each type has its own rate of occurrence and often tends to affect certain population groups sharing particular characteristics.

Sex, race, and other hereditary factors as well as geographic, age, and occupational differences— when added to differences in habits and exposure to certain substances—provide clues to the origin, and prevention, of many human cancers. Many types of malignancies are not necessarily fatal. Some grow very slowly and rarely spread; others can be halted by prompt medical intervention.

Although much remains to be learned about cancer development, extensive research has established that in some cases something identifiable is responsible for changing the behavior of cells and stimulating their uncontrolled growth. A single cancer-inducing (carcinogenic) agent such as radiation may trigger this response. While in rare instances cancer may follow a single large exposure, usually it is due to repeated low-dose exposures.

Most carcinogens seem to have their major effect in specific parts of the body, often related to their mode of entry and their sites of activation, destruction and exit from the body. But cancer in any one site may result from combined effects of several agents or several events. And variations in the body's internal chemical environment or genetic predisposition also play a role in determining the response to potentially cancer-provoking stimuli.

While the number of cancer victims has increased dramatically in the past 40 years, much of the increase is due to population growth. When changes in the size and age composition of the American population are taken into consideration, overall cancer death rates have increased only

FIGURE 6E

AGE-ADJUSTED CANCER INCIDENCE RATES BY SITE
FOR MALES: UNITED STATES, SELECTED YEARS, 1947-1976

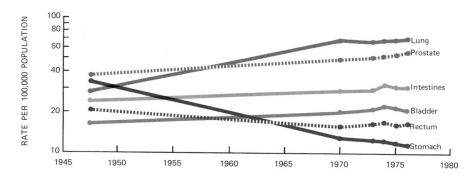

FIGURE 6F

AGE-ADJUSTED CANCER INCIDENCE RATES BY SITE
FOR FEMALES: UNITED STATES, SELECTED YEARS, 1947-1976

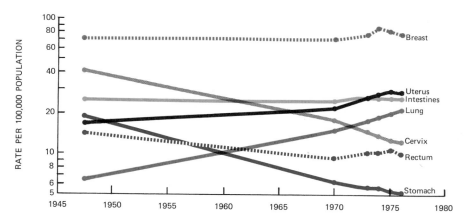

NOTE: All rates are age-adjusted to the 1960 United States population.

Source: Data for 1947-1948 are from the Second National Cancer Survey; for 1969-1971, from the
Third National Cancer Survey; and for 1973-1976, from the Surveillance, Epidemiology, and
End Results (SEER) Program, National Cancer Institute.

slightly for men since 1937 and have actually decreased slightly for women.

Also changed over the past several decades have been the patterns of cancer types and incidences for men and women (Figures 6-E and 6-F) and for whites and other races. Men have more cancer of the lung, intestines, bladder and stomach than women and have a higher overall cancer death rate—163 per 100,000 versus 137 per 100,000 for women. Whites tend to have higher rates than others of cancer of the breast, intestines, and bladder, but lower rates of cancer of the prostate, cervix, and stomach.

Cancer differences can be noted from one country to another. Compared to Japan, the United States has more cancer of the breast but less cancer of the stomach. Such variations in cancer types and death rates may be due to differences in hereditary, environmental and behavioral factors and/or use of early detection measures. The tendency of people who migrate to assume the cancer patterns of their new home provides some clues to cancer causes.

Risk Factors for Cancers

Among influences which have been identified as potential contributors to cancer development are cigarette smoking, alcohol, certain dietary patterns, radiation, sunlight, occupational hazards, water and air pollutants, and heredity and predisposing medical conditions.

Smoking. Cigarette smoking is responsible for more cancer and more cancer deaths than any other known agent. Not only do smokers have about 10 times the frequency of lung cancer; they also have three to five times as much cancer of the oral cavity, more than three times as much cancer of the larynx, and more than twice as much urinary bladder cancer as non-smokers.

Cigar and pipe smokers have lower malignancy rates than cigarette smokers except for cancers of mouth and lip for which their risk is approximately the same. The fewer cigarettes smoked, the less the risk. The risk also may be lower for smokers of filtered or low tar and nicotine cigarettes but evidence is limited and risk is still much higher than for non-smokers.

Smoking also can multiply—in some cases manyfold—the risks associated with other carcinogenic agents. Heavy alcohol use, associated with esophageal cancer, has a greatly intensified effect when combined with cigarette smoking. People exposed to carcinogens on the job may have much greater risk if they also smoke. The combination, for example, of occupational exposure to asbestos and cigarettes increases lung cancer risk 90 times.

Alcohol. Higher rates of cancer of the larynx, oral cavity, and liver as well as of the esophagus occur among people consuming large amounts of alcohol. Whether the nutritional deficiencies sometimes associated with heavy drinking increase susceptibility to the effects of alcohol, tobacco, and other carcinogens, or whether alcohol itself causes the damage is yet unknown. Contaminants that accumulate during manufacture of most alcoholic beverages may be the harmful agents, rather than alcohol itself.

Diet. A role in cancer development has been proposed for components of diet—and for some methods of food preparation such as pickling and charcoal broiling.

Some of the information about dietary causes is based on animal studies and may have limited relevance to man. Other information comes from comparisons of human cancer rates in different countries and among migrants from one country to another.

The typical American diet includes foods containing many substances added to enhance taste, improve color, and retard spoilage—as well as residues of food packaging materials, materials added to animal feed, and other chemicals.

Some of these additives may actually help prevent cancers—notably antioxidants and those that prevent growth of molds which can produce carcinogens such as aflatoxin—but others may have carcinogenic potential. Studies thus far have not been conclusive. But, because the number and amounts of additives were much less 30 to 40 years ago, and because malignancy can take that long to develop, careful scrutiny of the health effects of substances added to food is important.

Variation in rates of cancers (which differ greatly from country to country) may relate to differences in diet.

For example, people in Japan eat much less beef and total fat and more salt and pickled foods than Americans; they have much lower rates of breast and colon/rectum cancers, but higher rates of stomach cancer. These differences cannot be entirely genetic.

Among Japanese immigrating to the United States, rates for breast and colorectal cancers tend to increase while those for stomach cancer decline as eating habits become more like those here. Such trends are also found among immigrants from other countries. But the precise relationship between dietary differences and various cancers is still not known.

Radiation. A connection between exposure to radiation and cancer has been recognized ever since malignancies appeared in scientists and technicians who received large doses in their work with radium and early x-ray devices.

More recently, increased risk of cancer has been associated with radiation used for some diagnostic and therapeutic purposes. Because no radiation dose may be so small as to be risk-free and exposures are cumulative, some health professionals, while valuing x-ray procedures, have been working to reduce patient exposures. Much more can be done in this regard.

Other sources of low-level radiation to which the American population is exposed include those related to natural background radiation, nuclear weapons fallout, and nuclear energy.

Sunlight. Sunlight can cause skin cancer—and does among some people receiving large exposure, particularly outdoor workers. Americans living in the South and Southwest have much higher skin cancer rates than those in northern states. People with darker complexions are at lower risk. Protective clothing and sun lotions containing PABA (paraaminobenzoic acid) or other compounds that screen out harmful rays can help to prevent skin cancer, and premature aging of the skin.

Occupational exposure. Each year in the United States about 1,000 new chemicals are produced in commercial quantities. American workers are thus exposed to an ever-increasing number of materials that may have cancer-causing potential.

More than 200 years ago, an association between occupation and a specific cancer was recognized in the higher incidence of cancer of the scrotum among chimney sweeps. Since then, many substances have been found to produce cancer among workers in a wide variety of industries.

Occupational exposures can cause cancers which are rare in the general population—and, in the case of some exposures, can increase the incidence of a number of common types.

Working with asbestos without appropriate protection, for example, increases the incidence of the rare malignancy, mesothelioma, as well as of lung cancer. And, plastics workers exposed to vinyl chloride are at 200 times greater risk for liver cancer, four times greater risk for brain cancer, and two times greater risk for lung cancer than the general population.

Occupational exposures also may interact with other environmental hazards for a great multiplication of risk as in the case of cigarette-smoking asbestos workers.

Nor are hazards from industrial substances confined by workplace boundaries. Toxic materials may pollute air outside as well as inside a plant, endangering nearby residents. For example, angiosarcoma, a rare liver cancer linked to vinyl chloride exposure, has been diagnosed among people living near vinyl chloride polymerization and fabrication plants.

Moreover, contaminants carried home on work shoes and clothes can threaten families. Documented cases of mesothelioma have been found among people whose only known exposure to asbestos has been through living in a home with an asbestos worker.

Water pollution. Potentially carcinogenic industrial and agricultural wastes—including chlordane, aldrin, dieldrin, and benzene—are found in some rivers and lakes from which drinking water is taken. Although their concentrations in drinking water usually have been much lower than those known to pose substantial risk, such substances can accumulate in water supplies and may become concentrated in fish or shellfish. Their increasing amounts—and varieties—make updating and enforcement of water quality standards essential.

Air pollution. Air quality varies greatly from place to place within the United States. Air pollution comes primarily from automobile exhausts, the burning of fuels, and industrial activities. Pollutants such as asbestos, beryllium, benzene, and other synthetic organic chemicals are potential carcinogens, and several studies suggest that higher levels of air pollution may be associated with increased lung cancer rates. The extent of increase has not yet been quantified, but close monitoring of air quality is clearly indicated.

Heredity. Some cancers tend to run in families. Sisters and daughters of women with breast cancer, for example, are at higher risk for the disease.

But families often share environmental conditions and behavioral characteristics, making it difficult to determine how much of family clustering of cancer is really the result of heredity.

The significance of a family history varies from one type of cancer to another. Overall, only one or two percent of cancers are attributable primarily to heredity; in some rarer types, the percentage may be higher.

People with certain genetically-related conditions have a higher cancer incidence and are prone to develop malignancy earlier. One example is the predisposition of those with multiple intestinal polyps to cancer of the colon.

Cancers at Specific Sites

A great number of cancers and cancer deaths can be prevented through two strategies: limiting exposure to cancer-causing substances, and early detection and treatment before a cancer has spread.

Lung and urinary bladder cancers are amenable to the first strategy. More than 80 percent of all lung cancer and up to 50 percent of all bladder cancer could be prevented if people stopped smoking. Skin cancer also is largely preventable through avoidance of excessive sun exposure. Modifications in occupational exposure and diet may help to prevent other types of cancer.

Once cancer develops, many deaths can be prevented by early detection and treatment. For this, screening procedures must identify accurately people with cancer still in early enough stages to allow effective treatment. Available screening measures, more widely applied, could probably prevent a third or more of the deaths due to breast cancer in women over 50, most deaths from cervical cancer, and many of those due to prostate and rectal cancer.

Lung. Lung cancer, the most common lethal malignancy in the United States, accounted for four percent of total deaths and 25 percent of all cancer deaths in 1977. Approximately 80 percent of the 72,000 men and 23,000 women dying from lung cancer did so as a result of cigarette smoking. Early identification techniques—such as chest x-rays and sputum examination—generally do not discover lung cancer before it has spread. The elimination of cigarette smoking and occupational exposures to carcinogenic substances is the best approach.

Breast. Affecting nearly one in 13, breast cancer is the most common malignancy for American women. Although more frequent in older women, it does not spare the young and, 28 percent of the time, affects women under 50. Definitive prevention by any simple means is not available—but risk of death from breast cancer can be reduced substantially by early diagnosis.

Several screening procedures are available— self-examination (most important), examination by a physician, and mammography (a type of x-ray screening).

Most breast cancers are first found by women themselves rather than by physicians during routine examinations. Women should examine their breasts once a month. Particular care should be taken by those with family histories of breast cancer. For women still menstruating,

65

the best time is just after the period. Menopausal and postmenopausal women should choose a specific day of the month for breast self-examination so they are less likely to forget to do so. Although a lump, abnormal discharge, or size irregularity is usually a symptom of benign rather than malignant breast disease, a physician's examination is essential when any of these conditions is noted.

Periodic examination by a physician, in combination with mammography, increases the number of cancers identified early, before their spread.

Mammography may identify cancerous cell deposits too small to be detected even by careful physical examination. Among women over 50, it can contribute to reducing breast cancer death rates.

Mammography does use x-rays which, particularly in higher doses, may cause cancer, and frequent use of the procedure carries a risk which must be weighed against potential benefits. Each mammogram may raise risk by a very small fraction. It has been estimated that if, for example, a woman has five mammograms, her chance of ever developing breast cancer would increase from 7.0 percent (no mammograms) to 7.35 percent.

Colon and rectum. Cancers of the colon and rectum, which make up 15 percent of all cancers and are the second most common cause of death from malignancy, affect 100,000 Americans and lead to 50,000 deaths annually. They are particularly common between ages 50 and 70. Early indications may include rectal bleeding and bowel habit changes.

Premature death from colorectal cancers can often be prevented by periodic medical examinations, including use of instrument examination (sigmoidoscopy or colonoscopy) when indicated, to detect early disease amenable to treatment. People with family histories of colorectal cancer have special need for periodic examinations.

People whose diet is relatively lacking in fiber may have a higher incidence of colorectal cancer. The evidence that high fiber diets will reduce the incidence is scanty at present, but such diets are prudent and are likely to reduce the chance of diverticulitis and hemorrhoidal disease.

Prostate. Prostate cancer incidence has been increasing over the past 40 years, especially for black men. Four-fifths of cases occur after age 65. Not enough is known about causes to permit a strategy of prevention.

The best available alternative is early detection and surgery. Considering improvements in treatment over the last 15 years, the outlook is far better when prostate cancer is still localized at the time of diagnosis. Rectal examination by a physician is the most reliable method of early detection and should be part of every physical exam for men after 40.

Cervix. Invasive cancer of the cervix affects 20,000 American women and causes over 7,500 deaths annually. Rates of incidence and death have declined substantially since the early 1950s.

Risk of cervical cancer seems to increase with a multiplicity of sex partners, early and frequent sexual activity, and multiple childbirth.

Although the reduction in incidence and death rates began before such early detection measures as the Pap (Papanicolaou) smear were widely used, these measures are probably responsible for at least part of the continuing decline.

The Pap smear—for analysis of cells from the cervix—has greater potential for reducing cancer deaths than any other screening method now available. Smears—which can detect cells with cancerous potential before they become invasive—should be taken at periodic intervals: for three consecutive years beginning at age 20, or at the beginning of sexual activity; then every three years thereafter. The screening frequency should be increased for women using oral contraceptives or estrogen therapy, and in those found to have pelvic abnormalities.

Urinary bladder. Bladder cancer, relatively common in men, led to an estimated 6,900 deaths in 1977. About 40 percent of cases occur before age 65 and the malignancy is most common in heavy smokers and individuals exposed to cancer-causing occupational chemicals.

Blood in the urine is the most common early sign—but it may also signify other conditions, some of which are not serious.

The key to prevention lies in reducing cigarette smoking and exposure to carcinogens in the workplace. Many deaths may be prevented through early detection and treatment.

• • • •

The pattern of cancer incidence has varied widely—over time, across national boundaries, within subgroups in the population.

Only a small fraction of these differences can be explained by heredity. Environmental factors and factors in individual behavior appear to be the prime causes of most forms of cancer.

Therefore, many—perhaps even most—premature deaths due to cancer should be preventable.

Other Important Problems

Most notable among other problems posing threats to the health of adults are accidents (which have been considered in earlier chapters, and will be again in Chapter 9), alcohol abuse and mental illness. The latter two, as well as periodontal disease, deserve special comment here.

Alcohol Abuse

It is difficult to overemphasize the profound and pervasive influence of alcohol abuse as a cause of death for Americans.

There are an estimated 10 million problem drinkers in the country.

In 1977, more than 30,000 Americans died from cirrhosis of the liver—and 95 percent of the deaths were alcohol-related.

Alcohol is a contributor to several of the leading causes of death from age 15 to age 70, with direct responsibility for certain cancers of the liver.

It is a risk factor in various other cancers— and, rarely, in diabetes.

It is an indirect cause in many of the 150,000 deaths annually from accidents, homicides, and suicides.

67

Alcohol abuse also is a contributor to family disruption, child and spouse abuse, unwanted pregnancy, rape, assault, other forms of violence, job instability, economic insecurity, and still other problems.

Drinking during pregnancy can cause abnormalities in the fetus, leading to mental retardation and other defects. And special problems are presented by the combined use of alcohol and sedatives.

Chapter 10 will look in detail at the demography of alcohol abuse in the United States and strategies for its control.

Mental Health

Mental illness is a substantial contributor to disability and suffering for American adults.

The President's Commission on Mental Health has reported that three percent of the population— nearly seven million people—sought treatment in 1975 by specialists in mental health and one to two million were hospitalized for mental problems in that year.

In 1974, five percent of persons reporting limitations on daily activities indicated mental and nervous conditions to be the cause. Surveys note a large proportion of patients in the general medical care system have some emotional or psychiatric problem.

The Commission's report also indicates that, at any given time, up to 25 percent of the population is estimated to be suffering from mild to moderate depression, anxiety, or other emotional disorder.

Depression and manic depressive disorders are among the most severe types of mental illness in terms of prevalence, economic cost, and mortality. Of the 29,000 suicides recorded in the United States each year, more than 80 percent are believed to be precipitated by depressive illness. Severe depression or manic excitability handicaps an estimated two to four of every 100 adults at any given time.

Consistent relationships have been observed between mental disorders and factors such as sex, social class, and place of residence.

Women have highest rates of manic-depressive psychosis while men have relatively high rates of personality disorders. The incidence of psychiatric disorders is highest among people with lowest levels of income, education, and occupation. People in cities have higher rates of anxiety, mild depression, phobias, self-doubt and other symptoms of personality disorders, with only manic depressive psychosis apparently higher in rural areas.

There is persuasive evidence that appropriate treatment at the onset of acute psychosis can markedly influence its outcome.

Periodontal Disease

Disturbingly common among adults—and costly and difficult to treat—periodontal disease affects tissues supporting the teeth.

It is most often caused by bacterial deposits (plaque) on the teeth—and, in its most frequent form, gingivitis, produces inflammation of the gums, with redness, swelling, and easy bleeding tendencies.

Gingivitis often progresses to a more severe and destructive form of periodontal disease—periodontitis. At this point, bone and ligaments supporting the teeth are gradually destroyed and the teeth loosen or "drift."

In its most advanced form, the disease causes loss of teeth—and is, in fact, the prime reason for tooth loss after age 35. A recent survey found that more than 30 percent of Americans between ages 55 and 64, and 45 percent of those 65 to 74, have lost all of their natural teeth.

Careful and thorough daily brushing and flossing to remove bacterial plaque is effective in preventing and retarding progression of periodontal disease. Regular professional examination and treatment to remove hard deposits that form on teeth, correct predisposing factors, and repair existing damage are also essential for control of this disease.

• • • •

Many adult health problems today—it bears reemphasizing—can frequently be controlled by the individual. And the measures required are often not particularly dramatic.

An individual's risk of disease can be substantially reduced (or increased) by a few simple personal decisions with respect to smoking, alcohol use, diet, exercise, seat belt use, and periodic screening for major diseases such as high blood pressure and cancer.

The potential exists to promote substantial changes in the profile of disease and disability among American adults. But collective resources will have to be mobilized to assist individuals seeking to enhance their prospects for better health, as well as to protect them from threats not within their control.

It is encouraging that many voluntary organizations, large businesses, and community agencies have undertaken programs to help people adapt lifestyles for a healthier life. With a broad-based effort to provide this kind of support, we can anticipate impressive gains in the health of adults.

CHAPTER 7

HEALTHY OLDER ADULTS

Goal: To improve the health and quality of life for older adults and, by 1990, to reduce the average annual number of days of restricted activity due to acute and chronic conditions by 20 percent, to fewer than 30 days per year for people aged 65 and older.

If longer life has been one of society's most conspicuous accomplishments, there is compelling need now for another: a better, healthier life for older people.

More Americans today live to older age than ever before. Whereas in 1900 there were only three million Americans aged 65 and over, making up four percent of the population, now there are 24 million, composing 11 percent. By the year 2030, people 65 and over will number 50 million and comprise 17 percent of our population.

The death rate for older Americans compares well with that for older citizens of other countries, although we still rank behind countries such as Japan and Iceland (Figure 7-B). For all Americans over 65 the death rate is down from about 8,300 per 100,000 in 1900 to about 5,400 in 1977 (Figure 7-A). And for those 65 to 74, it has been amost halved— from 5,600 per 100,000 in 1900 to 3,100 in 1977.

But we have cause for concern.

The reasons for considering age 65 as marking the start of old age are mostly social, rather than biological. Aging is a subtle, gradual, lifetime process and there are startling contrasts in how individuals age. Even within an individual, different body systems age at different rates.

In short, age 65 does not mark the start of any inevitable uniform decline in physical and psychological functioning.

Nevertheless, the proportion of people with health problems increases with age and, as a group, the elderly are more likely than younger persons to suffer from multiple, chronic, and often disabling conditions.

Eighty percent of our older people have one or more chronic conditions and their medical treatment accounts for about 30 percent of the Nation's health care expenditures.

The long-term goal of a health promotion and disease prevention strategy for our older people must not only be to achieve further increases in longevity, but also to allow each individual to seek an independent and rewarding life in old age, unlimited by many health problems that are within his or her capacity to control.

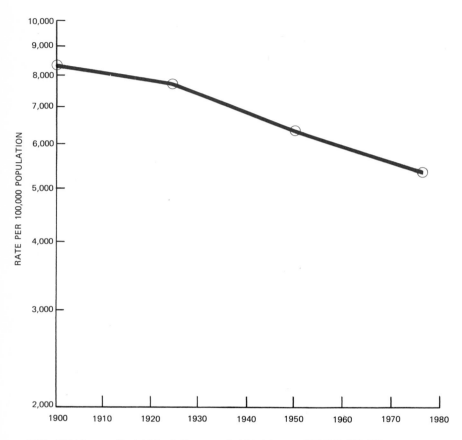

FIGURE 7-A

DEATH RATES FOR AGES 65 YEARS AND OVER: UNITED STATES, SELECTED YEARS 1900-1977

NOTE: 1977 data are provisional; data for all other years are final. Selected years are 1900, 1925, 1950, 1977.

Source: National Center for Health Statistics, Division of Vital Statistics.

FIGURE 7-B
DEATH RATES FOR AGE 65 YEARS AND OVER: SELECTED COUNTRIES, 1975

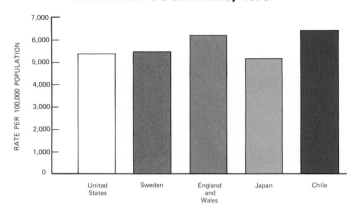

NOTE: The most recent year of data for Chile is 1971.

Sources: United States, National Center for Health Statistics, Division of Vital Statistics; other countries, United Nations.

FIGURE 7-C
MAJOR CAUSES OF DEATH FOR AGES 65 YEARS AND OVER: UNITED STATES, 1976

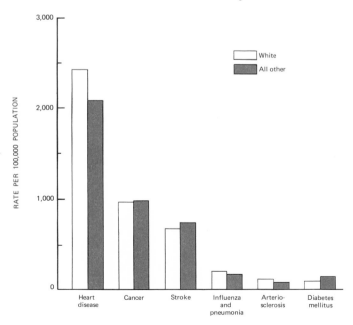

Source: Based on data from the National Center for Health Statistics, Division of Vital Statistics.

"Quality of life" is a phrase sometimes used to describe the latter goal. It is not something readily measured—but activity limitations due to illness or injury clearly compromise the quality of an older person's life.

Over the last decade, the proportion of people over 65 who have had to place limits on themselves, primarily because of chronic conditions, has fluctuated between an estimated 42 and 47 percent—only slightly less than half the 24 million elderly.

And the average number of days of limitation has changed little in recent years, ranging from 31 to 38 days per person per year.

But a large portion of chronic activity limitation stems from respiratory conditions such as chronic bronchitis and emphysema. Reductions in cigarette smoking among adults should lower the incidence of these conditions by 1990.

Moreover, a relatively small reduction in the incidence of strokes or a significant increase in persons protected from influenza and its complications could produce a noticeable reduction in activity limitation.

There is much that can and should be done to help make older Americans healthier and better able to function independently.

Subgoal: Increasing the Number of Older Adults Who Can Function Independently

As do younger people, older Americans hope for a state of well-being which would allow them to perform at their highest functional capacity on physical, psychological, and social levels.

Their greatest fear is of being helpless, useless, sick, or unable to care for themselves.

Despite a common misconception, most elderly Americans can and do remain in their own homes. In 1975, 77 percent had their own households—51 percent living with a spouse, 26 percent living alone—and 18 percent lived with someone other than a spouse. Only five percent lived in institutions.

Although the majority of the elderly are vigorous and completely independent, there are 45 percent with certain activity limitations—some associated with mental disabilities, but most due to physical handicaps caused by heart conditions, arthritis and rheumatism, hearing loss, and visual impairments.

Up to 20 percent of older people—from one-third to one-half of those with any activity limitations— are handicapped in ability to move about freely, compared with two or three percent of the 17 to 64 year old population.

Yet it must be reemphasized that only five percent reside in institutions—and many of these are temporary residents who are recovering from illness and will return to the community.

With adequate social and health services, a greater proportion of the elderly could maintain a relatively independent lifestyle and vastly improve the quality of their lives.

Disease-Related Factors of Dependency

Severe physical and mental decline in older people is not inevitable. While some changes with age are normal, many others can be avoided.

Although about half of the Nation's nearly one million elderly living in long-term care institutions are there because they were diagnosed as senile, that diagnosis is not always justified.

A mistaken diagnosis may be made because physicians and families may attribute mental decline and behavioral changes associated with physical conditions to senility, and fail to initiate appropriate and timely treatment.

Among the many causes of apparent senility which can be treated to reverse the condition are drug interactions, depression, metabolic disorders (thyroid, kidney, liver, and pituitary malfunction, as well as hypercalcemia and Cushing's Syndrome), chronic subdural hematoma, certain tumors, alcohol toxicities, chemical intoxications (arsenic and mercury), nutritional deficiencies, sensory deprivation due to social isolation or failing sight or hearing, chronic infections, hypoxia or hypercapnia associated with chronic lung disease, and anemia.

So numerous are the reversible causes of mental impairment that comprehensive diagnostic evaluation is often indicated. Moreover, there is growing consensus among authorities that even with irreversible organic brain syndrome measures are available to lessen patient discomfort, to slow or arrest deterioration, and to help the patient make use of residual strengths.

Emphasis needs to be given, too, to the potentially adverse effects of the many and varied drugs prescribed for the elderly. Surveys indicate that older people often have more medications prescribed for them than really needed—a danger which is frequently overlooked.

Evidence is accumulating to show that in older people the body's handling of drugs is quite different compared with the younger adults on whom drug clinical trials are usually performed. Moreover, the elderly, often suffering from multiple chronic diseases, follow complicated drug regimens that can lead to unanticipated drug interactions.

The mental confusion, and other untoward effects on physical health caused by drugs and drug interactions, can be minimized if older people have access to a continuing, well-informed source of medical care, with proper attention given to provision of only needed and suitable drugs and to patient education about drugs and drug effects.

At some point, too, elderly people are likely to need health or social system support because of social isolation, a dramatic change in their lives such as retirement, loss of a spouse, reduced income, or disease or injury.

Among the most frequent chronic conditions and impairments for older people in the community are: arthritis, which affects 44 percent of those over 65; reduced vision, 22 percent; hearing impairments, 29 percent; heart conditions, 20 percent; and hypertension, 35 percent. The elderly also, regardless of whether they are chronically limited in activity or mobility, are subject to an average of 5.5 weeks of short-term restricted activity a year. One third of this results from acute illnesses or injuries. Some acute episodes, such as burns, falls, or influenza and pneumonia, may be preventable.

Although most of the elderly are able to assess their own health status quite reliably, they may not always seek needed attention promptly. The problem may be due in part to unavailability of needed services, especially in rural communities. But it may also be related to fatalism, fear of confinement, poor transportation, or economic factors.

Communities would do well to develop outreach programs to find the sick and disabled in this population and help them quickly—when help can be most effective as well as most economical.

The potential of such programs has been demonstrated in a four-year study in Texas: the average number of short stay hospital days for mental illness patients 65 and over was reduced from 111 to 53 in a county that had a vigorous outreach and referral program; a similar county without such a program retained an average of 114 hospital days for similar patients.

Programs of geriatric screening can have great value in finding still-minor disabilities which, if left undiagnosed and untreated, can lead to severe handicap. Such conditions which are very much amenable to early detection and treatment include glaucoma, hypertension, some types of anemia, depression, hearing disorders, diabetes, some cancers, and over-medication.

The objective of an early detection program should be to preserve physical and mental health and enable older people to remain in their homes for as long as they wish and are able to do so. The screening should consist of systematic examination covering total physical, mental and social health.

Health surveillance and health maintenance for the elderly are most effective when a comprehensive, integrated system of geriatric services is provided at a single location.

One reason is that many of the conditions common among the aged are linked with other conditions. Diabetes, for example, may be associated with peripheral blood vessel disease which requires good foot care. But visual impairment, common in elderly diabetics, makes such care difficult and limited mobility due to arthritis may compound the problem.

Special diets may be necessary for people with diabetes, heart disease, or hypertension. Diets of elderly people are more likely to be deficient—in calcium, iron and fiber, for example—than those of the rest of the population. Taste and smell alterations in older people may diminish enjoyment of food, creating difficulties in satisfying nutritional needs. And absence of teeth, problems with dentures, and gum disease can make the situation worse.

Many elderly people, therefore, need a range of services—dietary guidance, eye care, foot care, dental care, and social assistance, as well as routine medical care. And these are best provided at one center.

Social and Psychological Factors of Dependency

Abrupt changes in social dynamics—and the elderly often face them—can create severe emotional stress and lead to serious physical illness, even premature death.

Older people are especially likely to experience drastic changes in family circumstances as spouses die and children move to other cities.

The stress of loss and grief is compounded by the absence of support which a family can provide. Stress is exacerbated still more when death of a spouse forces the survivor to change living arrangements and move to unfamiliar surroundings.

The elderly, too, must adjust to the change in status which comes with retirement—including the associated financial constraints many experience.

Although the number of older people living in poverty has dropped by 60 percent since 1959, due in large measure to Social Security benefits, still 14 percent of older Americans have incomes below the poverty level—a proportion higher than for the population as a whole (less than 12 percent).

Moreover, elderly blacks are affected to a much greater extent; 36 percent have below-poverty income levels. And women are constrained—with median incomes only about half those of men ($3,100 annually versus $5,500 for men in 1977).

Fear of the cost of severe illness may cause older people to conserve their limited financial resources. They select cheaper foods and housing, and make more limited use of preventive health services. Too often, the fear—let alone the reality—of financial straits prevents elderly people from leading the full and active lives of which they are capable.

Depression, a significant problem, may reflect loss of purpose in life. It is also related to presence of physical disease, loss of friends and relatives, other social difficulties, economic problems, and sometimes side effects of drugs often used by the elderly for such conditions as Parkinson's disease and hypertension.

Depression can be mentally and emotionally devastating, responsible for suicide or for seeming senility which may lead to needless institutionalization. It can exacerbate existing physical symptoms and may provoke new physical symptoms.

Many kinds of care and services are needed to deal with the complex, interrelated social, mental, and physical aspects of aging.

Limited dependency need not lead inexorably to total dependency. All who are functionally dependent, whether for a physical or mental condition, must be allowed—and encouraged—to do as much as possible for themselves, otherwise their abilities may deteriorate rapidly.

Absence of opportunity to choose among care and service options—as well as to participate in everyday tasks and decisions—is likely to produce apathy and accelerate dependency. The opportunity for choice not only promotes health; it also helps preserve individual dignity and sense of worth.

We know now what programs and services can help prevent deterioration, avoid needless institutionalization, and maintain functional independence.

They include programs for: safe and affordable housing; nutritious food availability through "meals on wheels" and group meal services; communication and transportation services, including telephones and escorts; recreation and education programs to promote enjoyment, challenge and stimulation; community centers to offer social opportunities; in-home services such as homemaker, visiting nurse, and home health care; ready access (including by telephone) to advice from a health professional; provision of eyeglasses, hearing aids, talking books, and large print publications; legal aid and counseling services; volunteer and employment opportunities to provide a continuing sense of purpose in life; and, not least of all, exercise.

Exercise and fitness for older people need emphasis. Aging is not—or should not—be a process of mere passivity. Nor should the obsolescent image of inevitable incapacitation be allowed to continue. Movement is part of functional living—and the quality of intellectual and physical performance is enhanced by remaining or becoming physically fit in old age.

Evidence for the viability of activity in enhancing function in old age is being developed through long-range studies such as those of the Gerontology Center of the University of Southern California. These studies indicate that people in their sixties and seventies and even beyond can retain, with carefully planned exercise, much of the vigor of their forties.

Older people can be more functionally independent.

Subgoal: Reducing Premature Death from Influenza and Pneumonia

In 1977 influenza and pneumonia together constituted the fourth leading cause of death among older people.

It may be true that for some of the elderly who are in late stages of physical and mental deterioration, death from these acute infections may not be untimely. Pneumonia has been called "the old man's friend" for the painless ending of life it may provide.

But many deaths occur in older people otherwise healthy and with much yet to live for. They can be prevented.

The greatest risk from the yearly influenza outbreaks occurs among the chronically ill and elderly.

A person over 75 is more than 10 times as likely to die of influenza as someone aged 55 to 64. Many of the chronically ill also are older persons. Chronic conditions which increase risk include: heart, lung, and kidney disease; diabetes and other metabolic disorders which increase susceptibility to infections; severe anemia; and diseases, including some malignancies, which compromise the body's defensive immune system.

For all high-risk individuals, annual vaccination against influenza is recommended—and those over age 65 should therefore seek the advice of public health authorities and personal physicians.

For pneumococcal pneumonia, we now have a significant development. This lung infection has been responsible for 54,000 deaths a year. Even with antibiotic treatment, it has been a serious threat to older people. The death rate has been 2.5 times higher for those aged 65 to

74, and 10 times higher for those 75 to 84, than for the population as a whole.

A newly-developed pneumococcal vaccine promises to be an effective preventive measure—particularly for special populations of the elderly, such as those in nursing homes and institutions where, because of close contact, disease spread is more rapid.

And prevention of both influenza and pneumococcal pneumonia can be vital for people with chronic lung diseases. Bronchitis, emphysema, and asthma are prevalent among the elderly and together constitute the eighth leading cause of death after age 65. The elderly with such conditions cannot tolerate well the added burden of acute respiratory infections.

Other Important Problems

Of American babies born today, three-fourths can expect to reach age 65; almost half will reach 75; and one-fourth will reach age 85.

Although many people are living longer, there appears to be a biological limit to the lifespan and it seems unlikely that, at least for the near future, any spectacular further gains in life expectancy can be anticipated.

While long life is desired by people in all cultures, quality of life may be even more important. And Americans now are witnessing the emergence of a new concept of aging.

It calls for the highest possible level of health throughout the later years—and, finally, dignified circumstances at the end of life.

It considers that a healthy society will view old age—and the inevitable death at its end—not as unnatural, but an integral part of the life span.

And it calls for society to learn how to help those for whom medical care can offer no more, so that death becomes possible without pain, discomfort, humiliation or financial worries.

A very real concern of the elderly is a prospect of being exposed to sophisticated technology that prolongs life beyond the time when it is meaningful and enjoyable. Nor can they view a busy, impersonal hospital as a comfortable setting for an individual who is dying. They have an additional anxiety: that the high costs of extended hospital stay place a heavy financial burden on surviving spouse or other family members.

Fears and anxieties about conditions surrounding death can be reduced.

When it becomes apparent that death is at hand, the health care system should be willing to accept the obligation to allow it to happen with as little pain and suffering as possible. The patient should be allowed to be in peaceful surroundings, preferably at home. Last year, most older Americans died away from home. When death is near, the greatest comfort lies in being in a home setting amidst the comfort and support that family members can provide.

• • • •

Many health problems of the elderly reflect past environments and lifestyles. The occurrence of heart disease, stroke, cancer, and other chronic afflictions may be rooted in earlier life.

When these conditions no longer can be avoided through preventive measures, early diagnosis and treatment very often can postpone death, avoid serious complications, and minimize pain, disability and emotional anguish.

Some health problems may be as much the result of basic human biology as of environment and lifestyle. Arthritis, diabetes, and some types of cancer, for example, may arise from changes in structure and function of aging cells. Even though knowledge is not now available to prevent these diseases, their course can be influenced.

There remain, too, many preventable conditions to which older people are vulnerable—including those such as influenza and pneumococcal pneumonia for which immunizations are available, and those caused or intensified by poor nutrition, lack of exercise, and other lifestyle deficiencies.

Thus, many measures can be applied to increase independence, self-sufficiency and quality of life for the elderly.

SECTION III—ACTIONS FOR HEALTH

FIFTEEN PRIORITY ACTIVITIES

Attaining the national goals described in Section II will depend on the development of effective strategies, many of which are applicable to several life stages.

This section is concerned with 15 important activities—grouped into three categories:

- key preventive services which can be delivered to individuals by health providers (Chapter 8);
- measures which can be used by governmental and other agencies, as well as by industry, to protect people from harm (Chapter 9); and
- activities which individuals and communities can use to promote healthy lifestyles (Chapter 10).

All are based on recommendations from a number of working groups recently sponsored by the Public Health Service and reflect the setting of priorities from a national perspective. It must be recognized that in some communities these priorities may need to be modified to local health conditions.

But developing measurable objectives within each of these areas, to be achieved within a reasonable amount of time, ought to do much to provide a better focus—and workable structure for both national and local efforts to promote health and prevent disease.

CHAPTER 8

PREVENTIVE HEALTH SERVICES

People are accustomed to seeking medical care only when they feel ill and ordinarily perceive no need for preventive health services when they feel well.

But we have evidence now that certain key services can do much to preserve health—and that people can be attracted to using them, with striking benefits, when they are offered.

Not by any means has every service delivered in the past in the name of prevention been efficient. Routine annual checkups, although traditional, have not been as effective in reducing health problems as the tailoring of pertinent screening, detection, diagnostic and treatment services to specific risks for individuals at specific ages.

Major progress has been made, however, toward defining what preventive health services should be delivered to the well population, designed for the specific needs of different age and risk groups. Proposed by various expert review panels, they have been modified as new procedures have become available and others found to be less effective.

While the proposals differ in some respects, they are notable for their similarities. What amounts almost to a national consensus on a core of essential preventive services has been developing. One list representative of the current view has been prepared for the Institute of Medicine of the National Academy of Sciences and is summarized in the Background Papers to this Report.

The five priority preventive services discussed in this chapter—family planning, pregnancy and infant care, immunizations, sexually transmissible diseases services, and high blood pressure control— are typical of the range of activities, the settings for delivery, and the blend of public and private, individual and organized efforts necessary for a well-rounded prevention strategy.

Other preventive services may also be important and some are discussed in Section II—e.g. testing for serum cholesterol levels or screening for cancer in appropriate risk groups.

The five included here are priority services with potential for substantially reducing death, disease and disability from problems affecting large numbers of people at earlier ages.

Family Planning

All pregnancies should be wanted. Any child whose birth is planned is far more likely to get off to a healthy start in life and to receive the continuing parental love and support needed for healthy development.

Yet, of the more than four million pregnancies a year in this country, one million are terminated by legal abortion. And of the slightly more than three million births, an estimated one-third are unplanned. It appears, then, that half of all pregnancies are mistimed and many are unwanted.

A large increase in demand for abortions has come from women aged 15 to 19.

From 1973 to 1977, reported legal abortions in the United States increased by an annual average of about 15 percent. In 1977, over 1,079,000 were reported—and over 332,000 of these were for women under 20. Although they represent 21 percent of all women of child-bearing age, 15 to 19-year-olds accounted for about one-third of all abortions and only 17 percent of live births.

But unwanted pregnancies are not limited to unwed teenagers. Each year, an estimated 300,000 married women have babies they say they do not want. In 1977, there were 190 legal abortions for every 1,000 live births among women who already had given birth to one child. The abortion rate for women with two children was 297—and for women with three children it was 358—for every 1,000 live births.

Unplanned births affect not only the health of children but also the social well-being of mothers. Early child-bearing interferes with educational attainment—and, because education is related to occupation and income, can permanently influence social and economic status.

The association of unwanted births with lower socioeconomic conditions and poverty also persists. And, clearly, having more children than desired can have adverse health and social effects on families.

Contraceptive Efficacy and Safety

Unplanned and unwanted pregnancies can be prevented with relatively safe and effective contraceptives.

Among the most widely used and efficient are male and female sterilization, oral contraceptives ("the pill"), and intrauterine devices (IUDs). Vaginal diaphragms, condoms, and spermicides (foam and jelly) are somewhat less effective but still acceptable and satisfactory.

The efficacy of contraceptives is determined by pregnancy rates among sexually active women correctly using a method. (Many methods require active effort by a woman or her partner and low efficacy can be due to failure to use a method consistently and well rather than to limitations inherent in the method.)

The established efficacy rates are: virtually 100 percent for sterilization; 98 to 99 percent for oral contraceptives; 96 to 98 percent for IUDs; 85 to 90 percent for diaphragm with contraceptive cream or jelly; 90 percent for condoms; 85 percent for spermicides. Periodic abstinence (rhythm method) is less reliable—about 80 percent dependable when used scientifically and conscientiously.

Actually, most people do not consistently use a contraceptive method correctly, and efficacies may be considerably lower than those indicated above. Often, incorrect use results from inadequate or inappropriate instructions given by professional providers.

Although not all long-term effects may be known for oral contraceptives, the relative safety of the various contraceptive methods is well established except for certain high-risk groups.

Among women under 30, the risk of death associated with the major birth control methods is eight to 12 times lower than the risk of dying as a result of a pregnancy-related circumstance. After 30, risk rises for women who use oral contraceptives and also smoke but remains low for nonsmokers.

In both cases, however, risk is less than that for women who use no method of contraception. Adverse reactions can occur in some cases with use of a particular method; when they do, a different method often is more appropriate.

The Non-Users

Although more women than ever before are users of contraceptives, including more than 80 percent of married women aged 15 to 44, 25 percent of sexually active unmarried women aged 15 to 19 never use contraceptives and about 45 percent use them only occassionally.

Reasons given by teenage women for not using contraceptives are that they can predict the time of the month when they are fertile, that they have a low risk of pregnancy, and that contraceptive services are not available.

Yet, in fact the services are widely available. Virtually all primary care physicians provide contraceptives or family planning counseling. There are also an estimated 6,000 family planning clinics in the country, a six-fold increase in the last 10 years.

What is apparently lacking is an effective outreach and information program to enhance practical accessibility and timely use of the services.

Where they are carefully designed and comprehensive, community-based programs serving pregnant teenagers have succeeded in reducing one of the problems of greatest concern—the rate of repeat pregnancies among adolescents. In Delaware and Baltimore, for example, programs which provide education, medical and social services, and infant day care have been reporting one-year repeat pregnancy rates less than half the national 25 percent average for adolescents. Such programs need more study but early results are encouraging.

Primary prevention efforts must also be more effective.

Making family planning information available at the earliest possible age is one need. Peers now are the most common source of information. Unfortunately this information may often be of questionable completeness and accuracy. In theory, parents are the most important potential resource for better information, and efforts should be made to improve both their knowledge and their ability to communicate the knowledge to their children.

Sex education courses should teach males as well as females the importance of assuming responsibility for practicing birth control.

However, only eight States and the District of Columbia now mandate some form of sex education as part of health education curricula, and only 39 percent of the Nation's school districts offer information on human reproduction and sexuality.

A major focus of primary prevention efforts must be on providing contraceptive information and services to all sexually active teenagers in a manner that is accessible, convenient, inexpensive and, perhaps most importantly, is effective in communicating with them.

Finally, family planning involves more than the question of "when" to have a child; for some people, the question is "whether." There are couples at high risk of conceiving a child with an inherited disorder. They may wish to consider that risk in deciding whether or not to have children. Alternatives available to such couples include adoption, artificial insemination, or conception and use of fetal diagnostic measures.

In some cases—such as sickle cell anemia, Tay-Sachs disease, and hemophilia—the important genetic characteristics can be detected before pregnancy through analysis of blood samples (carrier detection). Other genetic disorders, described below, can be detected during the prenatal period through amniocentesis and analysis of amniotic fluid, but detection of an abnormality may require a decision on an abortion.

There should be greater effort by physicians, clinics, other health providers—and by schools—to make the availability of these tests and alternatives more widely known.

Pregnancy and Infant Care

The chance that an infant will be of low birth weight and at increased risk of developmental problems, and perhaps death, is heightened by lack of early, regular, quality prenatal care, as noted in Chapter 3.

Although between 1969 and 1977 the proportion of women receiving prenatal care during the first three months of pregnancy increased from 68 to 74 percent, too many still do not receive care until the last three months—and the greatest risk is for the one to two percent who receive none at all.

From 1950 to 1977, infant mortality dropped from 30 to 14 deaths per 1,000 live births. While some of the improvement was due to greater availability of regionalized intensive care units for newborns, better prenatal services have clearly played an important role.

Maternity and Infant Care (MIC) Projects—part of a national effort to provide assistance to vulnerable populations—have consistently been associated with declines in low birth weight incidence and infant mortality.

In Birmingham, Alabama, for example, after the MIC project began in 1967, prenatal clinics available for low income pregnant women increased and the proportion of women receiving prenatal care during the first trimester rose from 24 percent in 1968 to 39 percent in 1978. Although direct cause and effect relationship cannot be determined, infant mortality in this area dropped from 25 deaths per 1,000 live births in 1965 to about 14 in 1977—and infant deaths during the first month of life went from 19 to 10 per 1,000 live births, a 47 percent decrease.

In Denver, Colorado, infant mortality was 28 per 1,000 live births when the MIC project began in 1965; by 1972, it was down to 17 and the incidence of low birth weight also had declined.

Prenatal Care

What are the important services needed during pregnancy?

They include thorough assessment of any special risks because of family history or past personal medical problems; physical examination and basic laboratory tests; amniocentesis where indicated; and counseling on nutrition, smoking, alcohol use, exercise, sexual activity, and family planning (Figure 8-A).

Through a prospective mother's carefully recorded medical experience and family history, it is possible to identify factors which may put mother and fetus at special risk for avoidable problems.

About 80 percent of women at high risk of having a low birth weight infant can be identified in the first prenatal visit, and action can be taken to reduce the risk. Without such care, as noted in Chapter 3, an expectant mother is three times as likely to have a low birth weight child.

Through family history, risk can be identified for several inherited diseases, including Down syndrome, Tay-Sachs disease, and metabolic disorders, all discussed in Chapter 3.

Women with histories of such problems as repeated miscarriages, bleeding, and premature membrane rupture are at increased risk for not having a live and healthy baby—but measures can be taken during pregnancy to reduce the risk.

Also needing more intensive obstetrical care are women who have congenital reproductive tract malformations or medical problems such as diabetes, hypo- or hyperthyroidism, heart disease or kidney disease.

Laboratory tests are important because they can confirm problems suggested by an expectant mother's family or individual history.

Women who tend to be more susceptible to toxemia of pregnancy are those with high blood pressure, diabetes or kidney disease.

Toxemia, which, when present, usually occurs during the second half of pregnancy, is characterized by rapid weight gain, swelling of legs and eyelids, headaches, elevated blood pressure, and loss of protein in the urine. If it persists, it can threaten the pregnant woman's life through complications such as convulsions and stroke—and lead to fetal death.

When detected, toxemia can be controlled by rest, sedatives, antihypertensive and anticonvulsant drugs, and correction of chemical imbalances. In most cases, it subsides after pregnancy but in some it has residual effects.

For women 35 and over, those with a history of multiple miscarriages, and others with certain genetic indications, amniocentesis should be offered. In this fetal diagnostic procedure, which is used at about the 16th week of pregnancy, a needle is inserted through the wall of the woman's abdomen into the womb to withdraw a sample of amniotic fluid containing cells shed by the developing fetus. Cells and fluid can be analyzed for chromosomal and biochemical defects.

FIGURE 8-A

PREVENTIVE SERVICES FOR THE PREGNANT WOMAN AND FETUS

	SERVICES	INITIAL VISIT[1]	SUBSEQUENT VISITS[2]
HISTORY	General Medical	•	
	Family and Genetic	•	
	Previous Pregnancies	•	
	Current Pregnancy	•	•
PHYSICAL EXAMINATION	General	•	
	Blood Pressure	•	•
	Height and Weight	•	•
	Fetal Development		•
LABORATORY EXAMINATIONS	VDRL	•	
	Papanicolau Smear	•	
	Hemoglobin/Hematocrit	•	
	Urinalysis for Sugar and Protein	•	•
	Rh Determination	•	
	Bloodgroup Determination	•	
	Rubella HAI Titre	•	
	Amniocentesis (for women over 35)[3]		
COUNSELING WITH REFERRALS AS NECESSARY AND DESIRED	Nutrition During Pregnancy	•	•
	Nutrition of Infant, Including Breastfeeding	•	•
	Cigarette Smoking	•	•
	Use of Alcohol, Other Drugs During Pregnancy	•	•
	Sexual Intercourse During Pregnancy	•	•
	Signs of Abnormal Pregnancy	•	•
	Labor and Delivery (including where mother plans to deliver)	•	•
	Physical Activity and Exercise	•	•
	Provisions for Care of Infant	•	•
	In Response to Parental Concerns	•	•

LABOR AND DELIVERY[4]

POST-PARTUM VISIT (including family planning counseling and referral, if desired)

[1]Initial visit should occur early in the first trimester.

[2]Subsequent visits should occur once a month through the 28th week of pregnancy; twice a month from the 29th through the 36th week; and once a week thereafter.

[3]If desired, amniocentesis should be performed at about the 16th week for women who are over 35 or who have specific genetic indications.

[4]Although not a "preventive" service, labor and delivery should be included in a package of pregnancy-related services.

Currently, about 100 conditions can be reliably detected by amniocentesis, including Down syndrome and neural tube defects. Neural tube defects also can be detected during pregnancy by a blood test and, in some cases, by ultrasound examination. Women with family histories of such genetic problems, or of multiple birth defects or inherited metabolic disorders, are at higher risk of having a fetus with a defect detectable through amniocentesis.

Also very important in prenatal care is the counseling of expectant mothers on potential problems for the fetus that may be caused by smoking, alcohol use, and poor nutrition, including referral, when necessary, to suitable social support services.

It would be difficult to overemphasize the need for seeing to it that nutritional requirements are met during pregnancy. There are increased requirements—especially for calories, iron, calcium, phosphorus and protein—and all the more so for pregnant teenagers whose requirements may be further increased by habitual poor dietary habits coupled with the accelerated needs associated with adolescent growth.

Maternal nutritional deficits have been shown to materially increase chances for low birth weight or stillbirth.

As early as 30 years ago, diet corrections—even in the last weeks of pregnancy—for women who had experienced famine conditions in the first trimester were found to help offset the potential effect of severe caloric deficiencies on the birth weight of their babies.

Although famine conditions do not exist in the United States, nutritional and socioeconomic status are linked, and many pregnant women, even some with incomes above poverty level, are not receiving adequate diets for normal fetal development. Providing an important adjunct to good health care are programs such as the Department of Agriculture's Special Supplemental Food Program for Women, Infants and Children (WIC) which gives dietary supplements and nutrition education at no cost for certain pregnant women, infants, and children up to five years of age.

Even before they become pregnant, women need to know about factors that may affect the health of their future babies. While providing information about risks of using cigarettes, alcohol and drugs, is an important part of prenatal care, many women are pregnant several weeks before knowing they are—and it is at the very early stages that the fetus is most vulnerable.

Early on, too, the fetus can be affected by toxic chemicals and infectious agents. Moreover, exposure to ionizing radiation above a certain level in the first week or two of pregnancy increases risk of spontaneous abortion—and subsequent exposure, especially during weeks two through six, increases risk of malformations and some childhood cancers, including leukemia.

Here, again, we need intensified educational efforts by schools, health providers, and the media.

The Birth Process

Although most women experience uncomplicated childbirth, about 20 percent have some problem during labor, according to the 1972 National Natality Survey.

There may, for example, be hemorrhaging, sudden worsening of toxemia, or impairment of oxygen supply to the fetus because of its position in the uterus.

Because these problems require prompt intervention, preventive care during pregnancy should also focus on the birth process itself and include education about childbirth and preparation of both parents, with underscoring of the importance of selecting a place for delivery in or near facilities that can be used to respond to emergency situations.

Recent technological advances promise improved capability for responding to birth process problems. Electronic fetal monitoring, for example, has improved ability to detect fetal distress and therefore to save the lives of many high risk infants. While the technique, if not used properly, may lead to needless surgical deliveries as well as maternal infections, it can offer significant benefits when appropriately used to monitor high risk pregnancies.

Postnatal Care

Once a baby is born, prospects for good health can be enhanced by a number of preventive services (Figure 8-B).

A simple blood test can be used to screen newborns for PKU (phenylketonuria) and congenital hypothyroidism. With dietary manipulation for an infant with PKU, and thyroid hormone medication for one with hypothyroidism, mental retardation and other problems that otherwise would develop can be avoided.

Routine neonatal care also includes intramuscular administration of vitamin K to prevent the bleeding which occasionally occurs in newborns, and instillation of silver nitrate solution in the eyes to prevent eye infection which might occur if the mother has active gonorrhea.

Prevention of Rh (rhesus) sensitization is a major advance. The sensitization can occur when a mother has Rh negative blood and the fetus' type is Rh positive. It can be prevented by administering a blood protein—Rh immune globulin—to the mother after the birth of an Rh positive baby or after an abortion or miscarriage. If the immune globulin is not administered, the mother may develop antibodies to the baby's red blood cells and the antibodies, during a subsequent pregnancy with an Rh positive fetus, may destroy the infant's red blood cells, producing anemia, brain damage, spontaneous abortion, or death.

Since introduction of Rh immune globulin in 1968, the estimated incidence of erythroblastosis fetalis (the disease caused by Rh incompatability) has dropped from about 4.1 cases per 1,000 births in 1970 to about 1.6 per 1,000 in 1977.

Despite its relative lack of public attention, the disease is still a significant preventable problem which affected 233 infants in 1976, 10 times the number born with congenital rubella syndrome that year. Yet,

FIGURE 8-B

PREVENTIVE SERVICES FOR THE NORMAL INFANT

	SERVICES	BIRTH VISIT	SECOND VISIT[1]	SUBSEQUENT VISITS[2]
HISTORY AND PHYSICAL EXAMINATION	Length and Weight	●	●	●
	Head Circumference	●		
	Urine Stream	●		
	Check for Congenital Abnormalities	●		●
	Developmental Assessment			●
PROCEDURES	PKU Screening Test		●	
	Thyroxin T4		●	
	Vitamin K		●	
	Silver Nitrate Prophylaxis	●		
IMMUNIZATIONS	Diphtheria			●
	Pertussis			●
	Tetanus			●
	Measles[3]			
	Mumps[3]			
	Rubella[3]			
	Poliomyelitis			●
PARENTAL COUNSELING, WITH REFERRALS AS NECESSARY AND DESIRED	Infant Nutrition and Feeding Practices (especially breast-feeding)		●	●
	Parenting		●	●
	Infant Hygiene		●	●
	Accidental Injury Prevention (including use of automobile restraints)		●	●
	Family Planning and Referral for Services		●	●
	Child Care Arrangements		●	●
	Medical Care Arrangements		●	●
	Parental Smoking, Use of Alcohol, and Drugs		●	●
	Parental Nutrition, Physical Activity and Exercise		●	●
	In Response to Parental Concerns		●	●

[1]Second visit should occur within 10 days or before leaving the hospital.

[2]Four health visits the rest of first year or enough to provide immunizations.

[3]Measles, mumps, and rubella immunizations occur at 15 months.

appropriate postnatal intervention could do away almost entirely with the disease.

Breast feeding. Emotional and physical nurturing are vital to an infant's health and breast feeding provides a way of enhancing both.

Until this century, breast feeding was the principal source of nutrition for infants during the first six months of life, the period of most rapid growth. In the 1940s about two-thirds of infants were being breast-fed but by the late 1960s and early 1970s, the proportion was down to about 15 percent. Recently, the trend has reversed; a 1976 survey found more than half of all mothers breast feeding.

Human breast milk provides nutritionally complete, convenient, prewarmed food for infants. Breast feeding also increases mother-infant contact, confers some protection from infectious diseases by transferring antibodies from mother to child, and helps women who have gained excessive weight during pregnancy to lose it.

Moreover, breast fed infants rarely are obese and virtually never develop iron deficiency anemia, the most common nutritional problem of American infants. If the nursing mother is healthy and well fed, fluoride and possibly vitamin D may be the only supplements needed by the baby. After about four months, a source of iron may also have to be added to the diet.

Commercial formulas are available and when prepared according to directions provide adequate nutrition but, in contrast to breast feeding, they are not regarded as the optimal food source.

Solid foods. Solid foods should be introduced with care—generally not until the baby is at least three months old. No adverse effects occur when solid food—and cow's milk—introduction is delayed until much later in infancy.

On the other hand, when fed too early, solid food may predispose an infant to food allergies, overeating, and choking.

In choosing solid foods, mothers should use nutritional value rather than taste as the primary guideline. An infant does not need sweetened or salted food and commercial baby foods should not be supplemented with extra sugar or salt.

New foods should be introduced one at a time, with each continued for a week before another is introduced. This helps identify and avoid food intolerances or allergies. Commonly, rice cereals are used first, followed by fruits and vegetables, and finally by meat. To determine the proper diet for an infant, parents would do well to consult a pediatrician, dietitian, or other health professional.

Immunizations

Because of vaccines, diseases that once ranked among the leading causes of death, particularly for children, now are regarded with less concern. Figure 8-C shows the change in incidence due to immunization.

But while substantially reduced as threats in most cases—and eliminated in the case of smallpox— these diseases still can be quite dangerous. Recent epidemics of measles and pertussis, and occasional outbreaks of diphtheria and polio, indicate that, short of complete eradication, reduction in a disease's incidence is temporary and immunization must be continually emphasized.

Childhood Immunization

Each of the seven major childhood infectious diseases which can be prevented by immunization— measles, mumps, rubella, polio, diphtheria, pertussis, and tetanus—can cause permanent disability and, in some cases, death.

The provision of protection against these problems has become a national priority. When polio vaccination became possible in the 1950s the Federal government moved to provide funds to State and local health departments for large-scale immunization campaigns. Similar campaigns were begun when measles and rubella vaccines were introduced. The combined Federal, State and local efforts were notably successful (Figure 8-C).

Yet vigilance in maintaining immunization levels has waned and large numbers of children are not adequately immunized. In 1976, more than a third of all children under age 15 were not properly protected—and the following year rubella cases increased by 63 percent, measles cases by 39 percent, and whooping cough cases by 115 percent.

In response to the low immunization levels and disease increases, the President in 1977 began a major Childhood Immunization Initiative. That Initiative reflects recognition of the need for a coordinated, broadly-based national effort to attain and sustain adequate immunization protection.

With the combination of safe, effective vaccines, public and private programs, and a reliable disease surveillance and outbreak containment system, infectious diseases can be controlled. In fact, complete elimination of measles is within reach and has been set as a national goal.

Although universal childhood immunization could eliminate a vast amount of suffering and permanent damage, barriers exist. Public interest must be maintained and parents must ensure that children are protected. The effort must be broad, involving not only public and private health sectors but also education, social services, and other fields. A recommended schedule is shown in Figure 8-D.

To help parents, health departments and schools should maintain outreach programs and educational efforts as well as programs making health services available on a continuing basis.

The poor are of particular concern since survey data indicate they consistently have lower immunization levels and higher disease incidence. Medicaid experience has shown that even where payment for preventive services is provided, there is no assurance that the services will be used.

On the other hand, neighborhood health centers, children and youth centers, and Health Maintenance Organizations have demonstrated that where services are provided in an organized setting, responsive to the needs of the population served, and coupled with outreach and follow-up efforts, preventive services may be used appropriately by all income groups.

FIGURE 8-C
REPORTED CASES OF MEASLES AND POLIOMYELITIS: UNITED STATES, 1951-1978

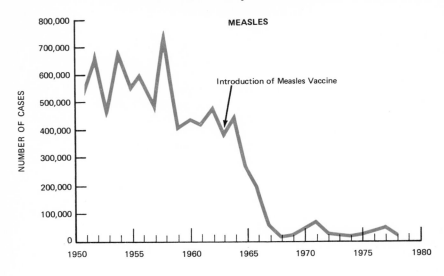

MEASLES

Introduction of Measles Vaccine

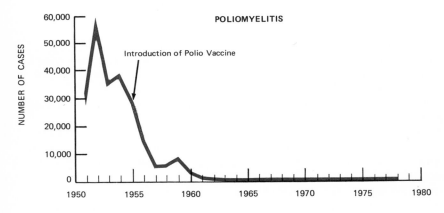

POLIOMYELITIS

Introduction of Polio Vaccine

NOTE: Polio incidence dropped below 1,000 cases annually in 1962. 1978 data for measles and poliomyelitis are preliminary.

SOURCE: Based on data from the Center for Disease Control.

Other Vaccines

Influenza virus strains change periodically, necessitating production and testing of new vaccines, often on short notice, yet vaccines for many strains have been successfully developed. An individual using the appropriate vaccine prior to the influenza season is 70 to 90 percent less likely to contract the disease. Annual vaccination is recommended for individuals determined to be at risk because of being over age 65 or with a chronic disease, especially chronic obstructive lung disease.

FIGURE 8-D

SCHEDULE FOR CHILDHOOD IMMUNIZATION

	Diphtheria Pertussis Tetanus	Polio	Measles	Rubella	Mumps
Age[1]					
2 months	●	●			
4 months	●	●			
6 months	●	● (optional)			
15 months[2]			●	●	●
18 months	●	●			
4-6 years	●	●			
14-16 years[3]	●				

[1]Immunizations beginning in early infancy are the recommended practice. They can be provided in later years, however, according to a schedule recommended by a family physician.

[2]Measles, rubella and mumps vaccines can be given in a combined form, at about 15 months of age, with a single injection.

[3]Children should receive a sixth tetanus-diphtheria injection (booster) at age 14-16 years, and every 10 years thereafter.

Source: Parents' Guide to Childhood Immunization, USDHEW, Center for Disease Control.

Vaccines against certain types of meningococcal meningitis are licensed and usable in case of epidemics. Research is under way to develop vaccines against other causes of bacterial meningitis, hepatitis, and several viral respiratory diseases of infants and young children but it will be several more years before these become generally available.

A vaccine with potential for reducing pneumococcal pneumonia by 60 to 65 percent is now available— and important because some types of pneumococci are becoming resistant to antibiotics. Use at present is limited to people facing greatest danger from pneumonia: many of the elderly, people with chronic debilitating diseases or sickle cell anemia, and those with inadequate spleen function. It has not been licensed for use in children under age two. Because the risk of dying from pneumococcal disease, acquired as a complication of influenza or otherwise, increases with age, it is likely that vaccination value also increases with age.

Sexually Transmissible Diseases Services

In 1977, some 10 million cases of sexually transmissible diseases occurred in the United States, 86 percent of them in 15 to 29 year olds. The diseases present significant health problems.

No vaccine is currently available to combat these infections but intensive efforts are under way to develop a vaccine against gonorrhea, the most common of the more serious diseases.

"Venereal disease" no longer is an adequate term since it has been traditionally limited to syphilis, gonorrhea, lymphogranuloma venereum, chancroid, and granuloma inguinale. Now, however, with other diseases known to be transmitted during sexual contact, such as two types of hepatitis, a more appropriate term is "sexually transmissible diseases."

The most common of those identified to date include:
- trichomoniasis—3 million cases annually;
- gonorrhea—2.5 million cases;
- non-gonococcal urethritis (NGU)—caused by organisms such as chlamydia and mycoplasma—2.5 million cases;
- genital herpes—500,000 cases; and
- syphilis—80,000 new cases a year.

While most of the diseases may cause burning, itching, and discharge, often they occur without symptoms and persons who have frequent sexual contact with different partners should be examined periodically.

Several of the diseases can lead to serious complications.

In young women, for instance, pelvic inflammatory disease from extensive gonorrheal infection or abscess in the pelvic cavity and reproductive organs is the leading cause of infertility and sterility. Gonorrhea also is a cause of acute arthritis in young adults.

Genital herpes—which is manifested by very painful lesions similar to cold sores or fever blisters—can cause severe neurological damage in an infant infected while passing through the birth canal. Such infection occurs in about 50 percent of infants delivered vaginally by infected mothers—and active lesions in a pregnant woman are an indication for a Cesarean section.

Although unchecked syphilis can have serious consequences, the availability of penicillin and an organized control effort have almost eliminated it in the general population. Certain groups, however—including homosexuals, migrant workers, and the poor—remain at high risk. The life of an infant with congenital syphilis is threatened when appropriate treatment is not provided.

For trichomoniasis, long-term consequences are not yet known, but no severe complications have been detected thus far. The consequences of infection by chlamydia, one agent of non-gonococcal urethritis, have recently been discovered to be eye infection and pneumonia in infants, and pelvic inflammatory disease in women.

Substantial difficulties hinder control of sexually transmissible diseases. Feelings of guilt or shame can make it difficult for some patients

96

to seek proper care. Professional and paraprofessional training related to the diseases has never been a priority in curriculum development. Some health professionals find it difficult to provide care in a straightforward, nonjudgmental manner. In addition, these diseases may receive less attention because they are most prevalent in groups without significant political influence—the young minority groups, inner city dwellers, and homosexuals.

Nevertheless, there have been successes.

After World War II, again in the mid-1960s, and once more in the mid-70s, renewed efforts successfully reduced the incidence of syphilis. Gonorrhea, which had quadrupled in incidence between 1960 and 1975, began to plateau in 1975 after a national gonorrhea control program was initiated with Federal funding in 1972.

One striking example of progress is found in a pilot program started in 1969 in Memphis, Tennessee, to control gonorrhea and resulting pelvic inflammatory disease. It focused on increasing public awareness and education about gonorrhea, expanding and extending the hours of clinic facilities, and increasing gonorrhea screening, casefinding and counseling.

By 1976, results were apparent: hospitalization rates for pelvic inflammatory disease were down by 50 percent from 1971—with the reductions most dramatic in hospitals serving predominantly young, poor women, the population mainly served by the national gonorrhea control program.

As the Memphis program indicates, the essential elements for controlling sexually transmissible diseases include education of the public, particularly adolescents, to understand early signs of disease and the kind of sexual behavior which increases risk; encouraging males with multiple partners to use condoms; screening high risk groups; treatment with appropriate antibiotics of all found infected; and identification and treatment of sexual contacts.

There is clear evidence that most important in attracting those who need the services are both the quality of the services and the attitudes with which they are delivered.

While existing programs are interrupting the transmission of syphilis and slowing the transmission of gonorrhea, many vulnerable groups are not yet being served. To approach them effectively will require not only the efforts of sexually transmissible disease clinics and investigators but also those of family planning clinics, private physicians, schools and employers.

High Blood Pressure Control

Controlling elevated blood pressure, which affects one in six Americans, is an essential if we are to reduce the 500,000 strokes and 1,250,000 heart attacks which occur annually.

Hypertension often begins early in life and becomes progressively more severe with age. It is one of the most important risk factors for coronary heart disease—and, for stroke, the most important.

Blood pressure elevation is more frequent, up to age 55, in men than women, but the reverse is true after 55. Blacks are twice as likely as whites to have it and it is more frequent in people with lower incomes and lower education levels.

In only about 10 percent of people with hypertension is there a known cause such as kidney disease or toxemia of pregnancy which sometimes may be followed by permanent blood pressure elevation. Excessive salt in the diet and stress are factors not yet completely understood; they may contribute to the development in some cases of what is called "essential" hypertension in the 90 percent of patients in whom the disease is present without any known organic cause. Recent evidence indicates that the hypothalamic region of the brain plays a role in the development of essential hypertension but more research is needed to clarify the role.

Although hypertension cannot be cured—except in the relatively few cases where a surgically or otherwise curable cause may be involved—effective treatments to control it are available. In most cases, medication is needed for a lifetime.

One problem is that because high blood pressure does not usually produce symptoms, many people do not take required medications, even when they are supposedly under medical care, because of failure to understand the significance of hypertension and its control. Some stop taking medication because they experience adverse reactions, as can occur with many medications. Yet very often an adjustment of dosage or use of an alternative drug more suitable for the individual can minimize or eliminate undesirable effects.

It is unfortunately true, too, that some physicians are not attentive enough to close control of high blood pressure for their patients.

Exactly how high an individual's pressure should be before treatment begins is not yet settled. But it is clearly beneficial when diastolic pressure—the second pressure reading, taken between beats of the heart—exceeds 105. Although research continues, it is generally believed that there are also benefits from treatment when diastolic pressure is above 95—especially when other risk factors for cardiovascular disease, such as a family history of the disease, excessive smoking, and elevated cholesterol levels are also present.

The risk of long-term use of antihypertensive medication in young people is unknown but thought to be low and certainly less than the risk of untreated hypertension. In some elderly people with only mildly elevated pressure, possible side effects may outweigh benefits of treatment.

Measures other than drugs that may be useful in preventing or treating hypertension are being investigated. Weight loss and dietary salt restriction lessen need for medication in some people and permit use of smaller doses for others. Exercise and relaxation therapy (biofeedback) can be helpful in some circumstances and are under study.

Because hypertension is a "silent" disease, a National High Blood Pressure Education Program was initiated in 1972 by the Department of Health, Education and Welfare. Targeted especially to high risk groups, it seeks to alert people to the high frequency and significance of blood pressure elevation and the importance of periodic blood pressure examinations.

And since 1972, as a result of education and screening efforts by government, voluntary health agencies, community leaders, medical societies, and health care providers, the proportion of people with hypertension who know they have it has increased from 50 percent to more than 70 percent.

Moreover, between 1972 and 1974, nationwide surveys indicate that the proportion of those with hypertension who received effective treatment doubled from 15 percent to 30 percent, and more recent State and community studies indicate that the trend is continuing.

For example, studies in New York (Westchester County, 1975), Illinois (Chicago, 1977), and Maryland (1978) have found, respectively, 43 percent, 59 percent, and 71 percent of the hypertensive population under proper care.

A longitudinal survey of a predominantly black area in Baltimore found that hypertensive patients whose pressure was controlled increased from 17 percent to 60 percent between 1971 and 1978.

The effects?

From 1972 to 1976, the age-adjusted death rate for all cardiovascular diseases declined by about 15 percent and stroke mortality fell by 25 percent. These improvements are almost surely due in part to better high blood pressure control.

A program in Milwaukee is one example of many successful community hypertension control efforts which have produced these gains. Initiated in 1974, the Milwaukee effort involved many community resources, including the health department, a medical school, voluntary organizations, an insurance company, the local media, industrial firms, and others. An important element in the program was development of a well-designed patient tracking system for thorough follow-up after community screening of nearly 200,000 persons.

And in Milwaukee, heart attack deaths in 1977 were 17 percent less than the average annual rate for 1971 to 1973. Stroke deaths dropped 38 percent in the four years of program operation.

Use of the worksite for hypertension control programs is especially rewarding. The occupational setting affords unique access to working people who may be not only at higher risk for cardiovascular disease but who are also less likely to follow through with appropriate treatment for hypertension.

As one example, a collaborative union/employer program providing hypertensive services at worksites for store workers in New York City has been successful in increasing, from 14 percent in 1973 to about 80 percent currently, the proportion of hypertensives whose blood pressure is under effective control.

The strategy for hypertension control entails using resources and services from a variety of sectors. And it also entails dealing with the kinds of individual motivation, lifestyle changes, and long-term intervention which are needed to address today's major health problems. But the results can be dramatic.

• • • •

This chapter has urged greater use of family planning services, improved care for pregnant women and newborn children, immunization for vaccine-preventable diseases, control of sexually transmissible diseases, and better high blood pressure control.

Each of these measures can improve the quality of life for many people and each is achievable with our current state of knowledge.

CHAPTER 9

HEALTH PROTECTION

The American environment today contains health hazards with the potential to kill, injure and disable individuals and substantially affect the health of entire communities.

Some estimates hold that perhaps 20 percent of all premature deaths—and a vast amount of disease and disability—could be eliminated by protecting our people from environmental hazards.

We have seen past improvements in protection— through better sanitation, better housing, better water—contribute greatly to increased life expectancy during the last 80 years.

But, during this same period, rapid industrial and technological development, social changes, and a larger United States population, concentrated increasingly in urban areas, have increased the complexities of maintaining a healthy and safe physical environment.

Nevertheless, measures are available to communities to provide better health protection.

Many communities and States have begun to develop health and safety standards to protect their citizens. And Federal laws and Executive Branch initiatives during the past 15 years have created an extensive Federal regulatory effort to help them.*

This chapter is concerned with five areas in which National, State and local efforts can significantly improve health and the quality of life for this and future generations of Americans: toxic agent control, occupational safety and health, accidental injury control, fluoridation of community water supplies, and infectious agent control.

Toxic Agent Control

Toxic factors in today's environment present formidable challenges.

During a lifetime, people are exposed, often unwittingly, to hazards from many sources.

---

* Health protection responsibilities are presently distributed among several Federal regulatory and research organizations: the Environmental Protection Agency; the Department of Labor's Occupational Safety and Health Administration; the Nuclear Regulatory Commission; the Consumer Product Safety Commission; the Department of Transportation's National Highway Traffic Safety Administration; the Department of Treasury's Bureau of Alcohol, Tobacco and Firearms; the Department of Agriculture's Food Safety and Quality Service; and the Department of Health, Education and Welfare's Food and Drug Administration, Center for Disease Control, National Institute for Occupational Safety and Health, National Institute of Environmental Health Sciences, and National Cancer Institute.

Although how all of these hazards interact is not known, for some it is known that their destructive potential can increase markedly when people are exposed to more than one.

Exposure Sources

Many of the agents posing new threats to American health are chemicals developed for industrial and agricultural purposes.

The growth of synthetic chemicals in the last 25 years has been extraordinary: more than four million chemical compounds are now recognized; more than 60,000 are commercially produced; about 1,000 new ones are introduced each year.

Some make their way into water and food supplies. While there are now substantially fewer dangers from contamination of drinking water by bacteria, the dangers of contamination by oil, fuel and organic chemicals are very real.

With the growth in use of chemicals for industry and farming, the Nation's waterways have become vulnerable dumping grounds for wastes from these uses. Food supplies as well are subject to contamination or treatment with chemicals in the course of growth, fertilizing, harvesting, processing and storage.

The dangers are demonstrated by recent incidents involving Kepone, polychlorinated biphenyls (PCBs), and polybrominated biphenyls (PBBs).

The insecticide Kepone, discharged from the Virginia plant in which it was manufactured, contaminated edible fish as it spread in unknown quantities to the James River, Chesapeake Bay, and the Atlantic Ocean. It caused serious neurologic and reproductive effects in workers exposed to it—and, in experimental animals, has caused cancer as well. It is no longer manufactured.

PCBs have been produced in huge quantities for use as plasticizers and insulation for electrical equipment. Not until tens of millions of pounds were produced and released into the environment was there any realization of how toxic and persistent these substances are.

Despite limited restrictions imposed in the early 1970s by industry to reduce production and use, high PCB levels continue to persist in the Great Lakes and other major waters across the Nation. In the past few years, PCBs have been found in tissues of humans and in the milk of nursing mothers. When fed experimentally to nursing monkeys, PCBs have led to serious injury of offspring.

Similarly, in 1973, the accidental mixing of the fire retardant polybrominated biphenyl in cattle feed resulted in contamination of food and livestock throughout Michigan. Growth deformities occurred in many of the cattle; thousands had to be destroyed. The health effects on the population which consumed contaminated food are still under study, but large numbers of people have been found to have elevated levels of PBB in their bodies.

Air pollution is another major source of hazard.

About 80 percent of Americans now live in urban areas where toxic gases or particulate matter pollute the air. Most of the pollution results

102

from combustion of fossil fuels by automobiles and in industrial activities.

Four groups of air pollutants are of major concern: sulfur oxides, including sulfur dioxide (SO_2) and sulfur-containing aerosols; carbon monoxide; photochemical oxidants, particularly ozone; and nitrogen oxides such as NO_2, NO and nitrite aerosols.

Increased air pollution has been associated with debilitating respiratory diseases such as acute and chronic bronchitis and pneumonia, and exacerbation of symptoms in people who already have pulmonary disease. Of concern, too, are poisoning from lead emitted to the air and the possibility of cancer from pollutants such as asbestos, beryllium, benzene, and other synthetic organic chemicals with carcinogenic potential.

Chemicals can be hazardous not only during their manufacture, formulation and use, but also during transportation and disposal. Community-wide exposures have resulted from accidents during movement of large volumes of chemicals across land and waterways.

And exposure problems are exacerbated by many community waste disposal sites containing large quantities of unkown chemical products. Many of these sites have been in use since the mid-1940s and their deposits may include highly toxic materials that can contaminate surface or ground water supplies or the atmosphere itself.

Leakage of chemicals from the Love Canal site in upstate New York reveals the risks to public health from chemical wastes disposed of before the initiation of regulatory controls. As chemicals began to leak out of the land-filled canal, concern arose about exposure for residents of homes built on the site. More than 80 different compounds have been identified, 11 of them known or suspected carcinogens. There has been a significantly higher rate of spontaneous abortions among exposed women. An association with congenital abnormalities is also suspected.

Several thousand such disposal sites exist throughout the country and close monitoring is needed to safeguard against harmful exposures.

Radiation is another environmental source of human illness. About half of all ionizing radiation to which the general population is exposed comes from naturally occurring radioactive materials in the water, soil and air. Another 45 percent is from medical and dental use of x-rays and from radioactive materials used for diagnosis and treatment. The remaining five percent comes from fallout, industrial uses, production of nuclear power, and consumer products.

Ionizing radiation from nuclear energy and medical diagnosis and treatment can, if there is exposure to large enough doses, cause cancer, genetic defects, and tissue injury. The entire population is also at potential risk as the cumulative dose of exposure to low-level ionizing radiation grows. Non-ionizing radiation, such as from ultraviolet rays and microwaves, carries lesser risk with single exposure, but the possibility of harmful effects is increased because total potential exposure is large.

Health Effects

It takes at least 20 years to determine full effects of many new compounds on human health—and health problems caused by some compounds in use today may not be known until the 21st century.

But it is clear that toxic compounds can have diverse, serious effects. They are capable of producing reproductive and developmental impairments, mutagenesis, cancer, chronic degenerative diseases, neurologic and behavioral impairments, and immunologic diseases.

Evidence for such capability comes from the experience of occupational groups exposed to greater chemical or physical hazards than those to which the general population is exposed. If high exposure causes serious disease, the same ill effects may occur in people exposed to much lower doses over a long period. For example, a single intense exposure to nuclear radiation produced very high rates of certain cancers and other illnesses among the populations of Hiroshima and Nagasaki, but radiation in much smaller doses also causes cancer over time in susceptible individuals.

Because successful reproduction and development are essential to healthy propagation of the species, agents that affect reproductive capacity or fetal development are of concern. Recent data show, for example, that men exposed to toxic agricultural chemicals such as Kepone and dibromochloropropane are at greater risk for impotence and infertility. In addition, more than 20 agents are known to be associated with human birth defects and many times that number cause birth defects in laboratory animals.

Of possibly even greater concern is the potential occurrence of mutations from exposure to environmental agents. A mutation—a change in the genetic material of a cell—can alter biologic development. If a mutation involves non-sex cells or is so drastic as to be lethal, effects are confined to a single generation. But if the mutation involves egg or sperm cells of either parents or fetus, the effects can be passed along indefinitely from generation to generation.

Probably the most widely discussed effect of hazardous substances is cancer. Statements that up to 90 percent of human cancers are due to environmental factors have received much attention but these estimates include as environmental sources such factors as diet, alcohol, and cigarette smoking.

Nevertheless, there are substantial threats from chemicals and radiation. The National Cancer Institute currently lists at least 20 chemicals and compounds for which there is epidemiological evidence of human cancer causation. Among them are asbestos, benzene, vinyl chloride, and arsenic. In addition, over 2,300 specific chemicals are suspected carcinogens, including some insecticides, herbicides, asphalt fumes, wood dust, and coal tar volatiles. They are believed to work through varied mechanisms.

Some produce mutations in the genetic material of cells which then reproduce unchecked; others may suppress the immune mechanism which usually destroys tumor cells; and others may stimulate the proliferation of tumor cells themselves. More than one mechanism may work at one time; the effects of exposure to single agents may be additive;

and concurrent exposure to multiple agents may be more hazardous than the sum of the individual exposures.

In addition to cancer, environmental agents can cause other degenerative diseases, including arteriosclerosis, heart disease, hypertension, emphysema, chronic bronchitis, kidney disease, liver disease, diabetes, anemia, neurologic and behavioral disorders, and immunologic diseases.

There is virtually no major chronic disease to which environmental factors do not contribute, directly or indirectly. Some of the most striking effects noted to date have been the neurologic and behavioral problems of workers exposed to certain pesticides, organic solvents, and inorganic metals.

Detection and Control

Protection against toxic environmental agents depends upon reliable methods of identifying hazards to health. Clinical and epidemiologic research has helped recognize harmful substances by finding unusually high rates of disease occurrence in certain population groups with unique exposure histories.

But disease generally occurs after a long latent period during which large numbers of people may be exposed to what will turn out to be the hazardous agent. Methods are needed to demonstrate biologic changes with potential for leading to disease— before disease actually occurs.

Animal studies provide one such method. With one or two possible exceptions, all agents known to produce human cancer also produce cancer in experimental animals. There is a popular misconception that under laboratory conditions any compound can cause cancer in animals. A study conducted for the National Cancer Institute found, however, that fewer than 10 percent of 120 common pesticides caused more tumors than expected when fed continuously to mice in high doses for 18 months, beginning in infancy.

Actually, animal studies have more often proved prophetic than not. That estrogen replacement therapy for women would increase risk of uterine and, possibly, breast cancer was predicted accurately by studies on several species of animals in the 1930s. Studies on quail in 1964 showed that Kepone could cause reproductive failure and nervous system disease. And studies on rats indicated that vinyl chloride gas would prove to be carcinogenic in the industrial setting.

A principal drawback to current animal testing procedures is the time and expense they require. A complete animal test of any suspected substance can take upwards of three years and cost several hundred thousand dollars. Several billion dollars would be needed to fully test the backlog of organic chemicals now in the environment but still untested.

Fortunately, encouraging progress is being made in developing rapid, less expensive tests for carcinogenicity and mutagenicity. Such approaches are designed to observe the short-term effects of toxic agents at the cellular or biochemical level.

They include tests for mutagenesis in mammalian cells, insects, and microorganisms; identification of any damage to DNA or its repair; malignant transformation of cells in culture; and chemical reactivity of activated substances. The rapid procedures can be used to screen large

105

numbers of suspected toxic agents to determine which to subject to more intensive animal studies.

When it comes to implementing measures to improve the quality of the environment, the challenge falls to all sectors of our society—individuals, health professionals, private industry, community groups, and government.

At the Federal level, several departments and agencies, noted earlier, conduct programs to identify, monitor, evaluate, and control harmful environmental contaminants.

Although these programs appear to have broad public support, their economic and technological impact can be substantial, and they are an increasingly common subject of debate inside and outside government.

Nevertheless, it is clear that the Federal government must continue to bear major responsibility for setting and enforcing pollution standards and for dealing with health risks related to environmental contamination. A strong emphasis on refinement of tests which can help identify potential new hazards is especially important.

State and municipal governments can reduce environmental hazards by monitoring the safety of air and drinking water; controlling use of ionizing radiation; providing adequate sewage disposal; requiring auto safety and emission inspections; and regulating the use of pesticides and other agricultural chemicals.

At the local level, individuals, community groups, and government agencies, including public health departments and health planning bodies (health systems agencies), can identify health hazards unique to a particular community. Easily observable effects on chronic diseases may on occasion be detected by community surveillance. Local education programs can help inform people about the hazards of toxic agents in the environment and how to protect themselves against them.

Although some significant environmental reforms have been achieved in recent years and the Nation's air and water are cleaner, environmental programs are frequently challenged and need stronger support.

Part of the problem in controlling environmental hazards is that they are produced as individuals or industries pursue diverse activities which have become parts of our daily lives. The automobile, electric power generation, plastics manufacture, and construction are all integral parts of present lifestyles and the economy—and all pose health and safety hazards.

The challenge is to reduce the hazards without undue sacrifice. But some changes in lifestyle may be necessary. Reduced use of automobiles is one. Eliminating waste in the use of energy is another. Reducing consumer demand is a third, and recycling is a fourth.

Because of the strength of competing interests, health does not always emerge as the top priority. But achievements of the past few years indicate that, notwithstanding obstacles, environmental changes can produce substantial health benefits.

Occupational Safety and Health

There are more than 97 million American workers—many of them exposed to some kind of occupational health hazard: carcinogenic agents, pulmonary or other physical disease incitant, or job-related pressures of noise, crowding, stress or boredom which can have adverse psychological effects.

Each year 100,000 Americans die from occupational illnesses and almost 400,000 new cases of occupational disease are recognized, according to National Institute for Occupational Safety and Health estimates. And the actual extent of occupational disease is probably much greater because the link between job and disease is often unrecognized or unreported.

Occupational exposures to toxic chemicals—as well as such physical hazards as excessive noise, radiation, sunlight and vibration—can produce chronic lung disease, cancer, degenerative disease in a number of vital organ systems, birth defects, and genetic changes that may be transmitted to future generations. Some hazards also increase frequency of stillbirths, spontaneous abortions, reduced fertility, and sterility.

These health effects are often linked with particular jobs. For example, workers engaged in manufacturing the pesticide dibromochloropropane have experienced an infertility rate twice to three times as great as for the general population. Examples of job exposure to carcinogens are noted in Chapter 6. Of nearly 34,000 chemicals in the workplace which have reported toxic effects, over 2,000 have been reported to be potential human carcinogens.

Yet, despite risks of serious disease or injury, most workers are unprotected. Worksite exposure standards have been established for only a few toxic substances.

Nine of every 10 American industrial workers are not adequately protected from exposure to at least one of the 163 most common hazardous industrial chemicals, according to a recent occupational hazard survey.

And now under careful review is a recent estimate that, if the full consequences of both present and recent past occupational exposures are taken into account, perhaps 20 percent of all cancers may be related to carcinogens encountered in the workplace.

Not all occupational hazards are found in factories or exposure to toxic substances. Work-related injuries kill about 13,000 Americans each year and affect nine million more so severely that they require medical care or are at least temporarily unable to work.

People in mining, agriculture (including forestry and fishing), and construction are six, three, and three times respectively, more likely to die from a work-related injury than other private sector workers. And work-related problems are reported by a wide variety of employee groups, including medical technicians, cosmetologists, flight attendants, dentists, air traffic controllers, and many others.

Health Protection Measures

Occupational hazards can be controlled by modifying work environments, patterns of job performance, or both.

Altering the work environment—plant, processes, materials used—is the most effective. Protection against hazards can be facilitated by requiring appropriate engineering controls, particularly as new plants are built.

For success, prevention strategies must rely heavily on employer efforts and support from employees, unions, and government regulatory bodies.

Worker protection may also require special protective equipment when other means are unavailable— and careful monitoring of workers exposed to hazards in order to ensure that safety controls are effective. Sometimes, however, conditions and circumstances hamper efforts to protect workers. Personal protective equipment, for example, often is uncomfortable and encumbering.

Effective protection also depends on the design and maintenance of equipment and proper training of employees.

It must be recognized that higher pay for hazardous jobs may lead employees to choose immediate financial benefit over long-term safety and health protection. And the concentration of industries with hazardous conditions in certain geographic areas, or their location in otherwise economically depressed communities, or their presence as the only industry in a community gives workers, in effect, no opportunity to choose a safer job.

Furthermore, development of hazard control technology has lagged behind the growth in industrial use of hazardous chemicals and sources of physical energy such as microwaves, nuclear energy, lasers, and ultrasound.

Even when controls are available, there are few incentives for employers to install or maintain them. Positive incentives that could be provided include low-cost loans, tax benefits, and technical assistance. Regulation is a negative incentive but occupational safety standards, important to preserving the health of millions of workers, should be strongly and consistently enforced.

It was recognition of the increasingly compelling importance of assuring worker protection that led to passage in 1970 of the Occupational Safety and Health Act.

The Act established the Occupational Safety and Health Administration (OSHA) in the Department of Labor, with responsibility for mandating and enforcing health and safety standards for the workplace and for educating workers about potential hazards. Scientific support for the Administration's work is provided by the Department of Health, Education and Welfare's National Institute for Occupational Safety and Health.

Pressures on OSHA are often conflicting, with some groups urging fewer and less restrictive standards and others requesting faster and more aggressive action. Clearly, enforcement of the Act, especially for workers facing significant health hazards—asbestos workers, textile workers, chemical workers, and many others—deserves high national priority.

Health Promotion Measures

Many firms and some government agencies have taken steps to provide worksite programs for promoting health through health education, physical fitness activities, and preventive medicine. Some provide screening for hypertension, high blood cholesterol, and heart disease. Some conduct or refer employees to groups to help them stop smoking or lose weight.

Encouraging results have come from a number of programs, and indicate the utility of establishing these programs for employees from the assembly line to the executive suite.

Some companies have become concerned about stress in and out of the workplace and are instituting measures to help employees deal with its adverse effects. Training in meditation and other relaxation techniques, and seminars on how to cope with stress at home and at work are examples of measures provided by some companies. Many employ company psychologists or psychiatrists, or pay for such services outside the firm. The extent to which such efforts actually reduce stress is still under study.

Beyond helping employees handle the pressures of work, a few firms try to modify the nature of the work. Some redesign jobs and organizational structures to try to make jobs more meaningful and fulfilling. For example, instead of assembly lines which require each worker to deal with smaller and smaller elements of a whole, some employers allow workers to assemble entire products.

Among other experimental measures showing promise are programs that allow workers to work in small face-to-face groups with a good deal of autonomy. The groups may be responsible for a given level of output but decide among themselves how to accomplish their goal, including deciding which hours to work. Supervisors concentrate less on giving detailed orders and more on making sure the groups have the resources they need.

Although they do not solve every problem of occupational stress, such measures have the potential to decrease job dissatisfaction and its costly consequences—absenteeism, employee turnover, alcoholism, waste of materials, sabotage, and plant shutdowns—and presumably thereby increase productivity.

Gaps and Needs

Despite increasing research into occupational safety and health, many gaps exist.

Inadequate data make it difficult to determine accurately the extent of occupational health problems and to measure the effectiveness of prevention efforts.

Because of long latency periods before disease develops, knowledge is lacking about the risks of the approximately 1,000 new chemicals introduced each year and how they may interact.

One problem in collecting statistical data about occupational exposures is the variety of ways in which people come in contact with hazardous agents—by ingestion, inhalation, skin contact, or some combination of these.

Another problem is lack of recorded information about the intensity, duration and combinations of exposures.

The difficulties are compounded by concerns for confidentiality—of employers over trade secrets, and of workers and occupational physicians over personal health records. Often, too, workers are not told the names, particularly the common names, of chemicals with which they work or simply do not know of toxic substances to which they are or were exposed. And when they do know, they may prefer to face possible health risks rather than the prospects of job loss.

Among critical areas that need study are the role of occupational exposures in producing birth defects and the special problems of women exposed to hazardous substances. Others include: occupational causes of respiratory disease, alone or in combination with smoking; the role of job stress and exposure to physical and chemical agents in cardiovascular disease; and the behavioral changes induced by chronic exposure to low levels of chemicals; the health effects of occupational exposure to such physical agents as heat and radiation and the interaction between these and chemical agents; and methods for analyzing thresholds of exposures to hazardous workplace conditions.

Finally, we need to learn what combinations of regulations and incentives work best to bring about changes in both employer and employee attitudes and practices to reduce known occupational risks.

That the work environment can play a major role in compromising health has been known for many decades. It is time now for substantially increased efforts to control known hazards, treat those afflicted, and develop techniques to identify and prevent harm from materials and processes not now recognized as dangerous.

It is time, too, to act on the recognition that the workplace not only should not contribute to physical or mental disease, but is also a legitimate and highly useful place for promoting health.

Accidental Injury Control

More than 100,000 Americans lost their lives to accidental injuries in 1977—nearly half of them from motor vehicle accidents, the rest from falls, burns, poisonings and other causes. In 1977, too, 65 million people suffered non-fatal accidental injuries, requiring medical treatment—and in terms of damage, injury and lost productivity, the estimated cost of accidents in 1977 was $62 billion.

The leading cause of death beween ages one and 44, accidents account for roughly 50 percent of fatalities for those 15 to 24. But the highest death rate for accidents occurs among the elderly whose risk of fatal injury is nearly double that of adolescents and young adults.

Educational approaches advocating changes in behavior have been generally ineffective in preventing accidents among those at highest risk—young children, teenage males, problem drinkers, and the elderly.

More effective measures involve changing the manmade environment to reduce risk for those unable to take adequate precautions. Such efforts are certainly not unprecedented. Examples include insulated tools, childproof medication containers, lead-free paints, and automobile airbags.

Motor Vehicle Accidents

Highway accidents in 1977 killed 49,000 people and led to 1,800,000 disabling injuries. The total cost, as estimated by the Department of Transportation was more than $43 billion.

Teenagers and young adults—the 15 to 24 year olds—have the highest motor vehicle death rate of any group, accounting for one-third of all motor vehicle deaths.

Like many other types of accidents, motor vehicle crashes traditionally have been blamed on human error, and prevention strategies have consisted primarily of driver education programs. But more recently, injury control experts have identified a range of factors in vehicle collisions which occur with imbalances between the demand of the highway system, the characteristics of individual vehicles, and the age and other characteristics of the driver.

Moreover, it appears that injuries often can be prevented or reduced even when collisions occur. A number of preventive strategies emerge—some aimed at preventing collision, others at minimizing their consequences.

Many collisions obviously can be prevented by reducing vehicle numbers and miles traveled by automobile through encouraging people to travel by air, rail or bus—all safer modes of transportation.

Similarly, lower speed limits, if observed, would reduce both the number and severity of crashes—and, for several years after it was imposed in 1974, the national 55 mph speed limit saved an estimated 4,000 to 5,000 lives each year.

The greatest risk factor for fatal accidents is driver alcohol use. In about 50 percent of drivers involved in fatal crashes, blood alcohol levels have been found to be excessive. Although driver education and strict penalties such as mandatory license suspension have the potential to reduce alcohol-related accidents, those measures have not been very effective to date. Clearly important are the general preventive measures to reduce problem drinking discussed in Chapter 10.

Vehicle design is another major factor in highway injury and death. To reduce crash impact on driver and passengers, automobile bumpers, front ends, and steering columns can be designed to absorb energy. Passenger compartments can be better designed to withstand accidents, with protruding knobs and handles eliminated and hard surfaces padded. Although some of these design features have been adopted, most cars are not designed to fully protect occupants from injury in crashes that occur at legal let alone high speeds.

Combined lap and shoulder belts can almost halve the likelihood of serious injury or death, and although all passenger vehicles sold in the United States are equipped with seat belts, fewer than 20 percent of drivers use them.

Current Federal law requires that by 1983 all new cars contain devices that automatically protect front seat passengers in frontal collisions. The devices—such as airbags and belts that are automatically positioned when the car door is closed— promise substantial protection. The National Highway Traffic Safety Administration recently reported a fatality rate for one type of car equipped with automatic belts only half that for the same type equipped with conventional safety belts.

If no child died in an automobile accident, the death rate for children could be reduced by fully one-fifth. Now, about 1,000 youngsters under age five die, and more than 50,000 suffer serious injury each year.

A number of devices specially designed for children provide the best protection. Their use should begin with a newborn's trip home from the hospital. In the absence of the special restraints, adult seat belts are better than nothing. Beyond reducing risk of serious injury or death, use of restraints may help ensure that children acquire a lifelong habit of wearing protection.

Yet—in the face of evidence showing their effectiveness—a 1974 survey by the Insurance Institute for Highway Safety found proper restraints in use for only seven percent of almost 9,000 passengers under age 10.

Because efforts to convince most people to use child restraints have not been successful, it is important that passive protection devices be developed with children in mind.

An additional action is suggested by the success that changing school hours to non-rush hours has had in some European countries in helping to reduce automobile-related deaths for children.

The motorcycle helmet has proved to be the most effective device for protecting riders from death or serious injury in a collision. Riders using safety helmets have less than half as many moderate to severe head injuries and three to nine times fewer fatal head injuries.

Although helmets are worn 90 to 99 percent of the time in States which require them, they are used less than 60 percent of the time in States which have repealed such laws.

Motorcyclists often contend that helmet laws infringe on personal liberties—and opponents of mandatory laws argue that since other people usually are not endangered, the individual motorcyclist should be allowed personal responsibility for risk.

But the high costs of disabling and fatal injuries, the burdens on families, and the demands on medical care resources are borne by society as a whole. And society has a legitimate concern for protecting the individual.

In Colorado, Kansas and South Dakota—states for which pre- and post-repeal crash data are available—head injuries rose and fatal head injuries doubled after helmet laws were repealed.

The interstate highway system has achieved a halving of death rates compared to all other roads by eliminating crash-precipitating features such as sharp curves, steep grades, blind intersections, uncontrolled access, and lack of physical separation between opposing traffic lanes.

Other measures for preventing death and injury include removing fixed objects or shielding such structures as bridge abutments with energy-absorbing barriers, locating essential signs and poles at sufficient distance from traffic, and designing guardrails to guide vehicles away from hazards.

The importance of these measures is underlined by the fact that almost half of all motor vehicle deaths involve only one vehicle.

Firearms

Second only to motor vehicles as a cause of fatal injury, firearms in 1977 claimed some 32,000 lives. About 13,000 deaths were homicides; 2,000 resulted from firearm accidents; 16,000 people took their own lives with firearms; the remaining 1,000 deaths were of undetermined cause. Estimates of non-fatal firearm injuries—many of them permanently disabling—range from 18,000 to more than 100,000.

Although homicides committed with firearms have recently declined after a 10-year period during which the rate doubled, FBI statistics show that in 1976 firearms were used in about 63 percent of homicides, almost half of which were committed with handguns.

Meanwhile, firearm suicides have risen, increasing by 25 percent between 1970 and 1976, while suicides by other methods increased three percent.

Measures that could reduce risk of firearm deaths and injuries range from encouraging safer storage and use to a ban on private ownership.

Evidence from England suggests that prohibiting possession of handguns would reduce the number of deaths and injuries, particularly those unrelated to criminal assaults. Both assaults and suicide attempts are less likely to be fatal without firearms—and firearm accidents would decrease.

About 20 percent of American households contain a handgun. Even if reducing handgun availability did not substantially reduce the number of murders committed during violent crimes, it would likely reduce both accidental deaths and murders of passion involving family members and acquaintances.

For those who feel compelled to keep handguns, certain safety measures can be useful—security locks, use of non-lethal (wax) bullets, and weapon storage in a location separate from ammunition and inaccessible to children.

Falls

Fifteen thousand Americans are killed and about 14 million are injured each year by falls.

Fatal falls occur primarily in the home but are also a prominent cause of work-injury deaths, especially among construction workers. People over age 75 account for about 60 percent of the deaths resulting from falls and an even greater proportion of the hospital days and disability.

Preventing such deaths and injuries requires preventing the falls themselves by attention to safer walking surfaces and footgear, better illumination, handrails, and window guards—or reducing the potential for injury by minimizing the distances people fall (lower beds for the elderly) or modifying the surfaces they fall against (softer floors, rounded edges and corners on furniture).

Substantial reductions in injuries from falls can be achieved through elementary and inexpensive changes in housing and furniture design.

Burns

Each year more than a million Americans are burned, 60,000 severely enough to require hospitalization. About 5,000 deaths result from fires—predominantly house fires—and an additional 2,500 are from other burns such as electrical and scalds.

Fifty-six percent of fatal residential fires—and a substantial number of burn injuries—are cigarette-related, often due to smoking in bed. Even in the non-fatal incidents, the consequences are often tragic: painful recovery, disfigurement, and disability.

Many deaths and injuries from residential fires could be prevented through a number of measures: effective fire or smoke detection systems; less flammable furnishings and structural materials; buildings designed for ease of escape; developing and practicing fire evacuation procedures; and less smoking.

Deaths and injuries from ignited clothing have been greatly reduced in the past decade, partly through changes in fabrics and styles, but the problem still warrants attention. Other preventive measures are available but seldom used: matches that burn with less heat and go out when dropped, and fabrics whose weave, finish, composition or chemical treatment makes them less likely to ignite, melt or burn.

Scalds, which cause about 40 percent of hospital admissions for burns, often occur in showers and bathtubs. They could be prevented if water heaters in homes, nursing homes, dormitories, and hotels were modified with automated cut-offs so water temperatures remain below those likely to scald.

A recent study for the Consumer Product Safety Commission indicates that this approach, even though it requires larger hot water storage facilities, saves both money and energy.

Poisoning

Once a leading cause of death for young children, poisoning has decreased significantly as paint lead content has been reduced and drugs and household products have been packaged in childproof containers.

Of 4,000 fatal poisonings in 1977, less than one percent involved children under five. Even as the number of children increased between 1968 and 1976, childhood deaths from poisoning dropped from 284 in 1968 to 105 in 1976.

Still, some two million ingestions of potentially dangerous substances by American children come to the attention of health professionals every year.

Poison Control Centers, now active in a number of localities, provide immediate information on poison antidotes and other emergency measures. Helpful precautionary measures include storing toxic substances separately from food supplies, ensuring that safety caps are fastened, and refraining from introducing medicine to children as "candy."

Currently, treatment of lead poisoning makes use of chemicals that bind to the metal in the body and help in its removal.

But more important is primary prevention of potentially lethal lead poisoning by removal of airborne lead from the environment and rehabilitation of old housing with lead-free paint. Public health screening of high-risk children is important to prevention of adverse health effects, since lead poisoning is usually asymptomatic.

Drug Reactions

Some 70,000 prescription drugs (with 2,000 individual ingredients) are now on the market, along with 200,000 over-the-counter preparations. Each year 15 to 20 new chemical entities are introduced. In 1977, 1.4 billion prescriptions were filled at a cost of about $8 billion.

Adverse reactions—ranging from moderate rashes or nausea to birth defects or death—can occur with almost any drug. For some drugs, reactions are frequent enough to warrant warning labels.

The potential for adverse reactions, coupled with the volume and frequency of drug use, requires the Food and Drug Administration to oversee regular premarket screening and testing for user protection.

Product-Related Accidents

A broad range of consumer products used at home or in the workplace can cause injury, either because of faulty construction or inappropriate and careless use.

In 1976, product-related accidents caused about 30,000 deaths and 37 million injuries, according to Consumer Product Safety Commission estimates.

Among the leading causes of injuries were glass, bicycles, skateboards, nails, knives, playground equipment, furniture, and construction and flooring materials.

Measures to reduce injuries and deaths can start with product design and engineering standards—and the education of those developing the designs and standards. They can include improved construction and packaging; testing and development of protective devices; inspection procedures to ensure safety prior to marketing or operation; and better instruction of operators of machinery as well as more complete and clear information provided for consumers and users.

Because unsafe toys, electrical devices, and home swimming pools injure many chidren, toys with sharp edges or small and swallowable parts should be discarded, electrical outlets should be covered, and swimming pools fenced.

Increased protection for children requires better surveillance of injuries so their causes can be clearly understood and preventive measures applied. It also requires teaching safe behavior and providing barriers that separate children from as many hazards as possible.

Recreational Accidents

The population at risk for recreational accidents has grown steadily as the amount of leisure time available to Americans has increased.

According to the National Safety Council, accidents other than motor vehicle, work and home accidents caused approximately 21,500 deaths in 1976, with most occurring in recreational or leisure settings.

Disabling injuries in that year numbered some 2,700,000 and about 100,000 sports team injuries were serious enough to require medical attention. Some 7,000 drownings also occur each year, mostly during water sports such as swimming and boating.

Safety measures can help. Children can be taught to float and swim at an early age and should learn water safety measures. Adults can avoid water sports when intoxicated (in almost one-third of adult drownings, there are high blood levels of alcohol). Young people participating in team sports can be taught safety measures and ways to prevent injuries as part of their training. Better protective equipment can be developed. Football helmets, for example, which caused 12 percent of all injuries sustained by 9,000 high school players, should be designed to reduce injuries to other players.

Modification of surroundings can help in some cases. Again, in football it is estimated that seven percent of hospitalized players are injured as the result of striking a fixed obstacle outside the playing field and that 95 percent of such injuries could be prevented by establishing an obstacle-free zone around the playing field.

Much can be done to prevent unnecessary injuries annually suffered by Americans.

Fluoridation of Community Water Supplies

With tooth decay affecting 95 percent of Americans, it is the most common health problem, costing an estimated $2 billion yearly for treatment. Adverse consequences include pain, infection and tooth loss.

Fluoridation is one of the most effective—and cost-effective—preventive measures known. By making teeth less susceptible to decay through increasing resistance to the action of bacteria-produced acid (it may have an antibacterial effect as well), optimal level fluoridation of drinking water can prevent 65 percent of decay that would otherwise occur. And it can do so for 10 to 40 cents per person per year, depending upon the size of the community.

Currently, less than half of Americans have access to fluoridated water. About a third are served by fluoride-deficient community water systems. An additional 35 to 40 million are on individual (noncommunal) water systems with undetermined fluoride content.

Where community water supplies are not fluoridated or where there is no central source of drinking water, as in many rural areas, other means may be used. In some localities, school drinking water is fluoridated—a help in reducing decay but less effective than community-wide fluoridation since it does not reach pre-school children and is not available to any child when school is not in session.

Fluoride mouth rinses are effective but require regular, continued use for maximum benefits. In carefully controlled clinical studies, fluoride rinsing has produced 35 percent decay reduction.

If dietary fluoride supplements are given conscientiously from birth on a daily basis, the protection against decay approaches that of water fluoridation.

Fluoride applied directly to teeth twice a year by a dental profession-al in a school program or dentist's office also is effective as is daily use of an appropriately formulated fluoride toothpaste.

But none of these approaches is as effective or economical as fluori-dated drinking water.

Part of the delay in fluoridation of community water supplies stems from concerns of some groups that it may pose a hazard to health. But substantial research over the past 35 years has produced no evidence to support this concern.

It is important that every community ensure provision of fluoridated drinking water for its citizens.

Infectious Agent Control

Some 291 million illnesses from infectious disease occurred in the United States in 1975—more than one for every person. Because of them, each year at least 156 million work days are lost and the cost for treatment and lost productivity is estimated at $24 billion annually.

In a typical year, the Center for Disease Control investigates, upon request, about 1,700 outbreaks of infectious diseases throughout the country.

Most of the deaths and illnesses related to infectious diseases are due to the viral, bacterial and other microbial agents of influenza, pneumo-nia, the common cold, urinary tract infections, gastroenteritis, hepatitis, childhood infectious diseases, sexually transmissible diseases, tuberculo-sis, and hospital-acquired infections.

There has been substantial success, as noted earlier, in minimizing the infectious diseases as threats to life. In 1977, only influenza and pneu-monia together continued to rank as one of the 10 leading causes of death.

But new diseases appear and even familiar diseases may change peri-odically, making existing protective measures ineffective.

Legionnaires' disease is an example of a newly identified infection. The emergence of strains of gonococcal bacteria resistant to penicillin, and the periodic shifts in strains and virulence of influenza viruses, are examples of changes in familiar diseases.

These changes demand close monitoring and surveillance of infec-tious disease incidence.

Surveillance—a basic tactic for disease control—requires four activi-ties.

- finding cases of disease or significant exposures through the ef-forts of physicians and other health workers;
- reporting cases to a responsible health authority, generally a public health official—traditionally done by physicians, but now also done by schools and industries;
- analyzing and interpreting the reported information to determine its implications; and
- responding appropriately to the interpreted information with measures to control the source of the problem.

Examples of response measures include an immunization campaign in the face of a polio outbreak, closing a restaurant found to be serving contaminated food, and providing substitute water supplies until a polluted source can be purified.

Today, about five percent of all patients admitted to hospitals acquire an infection while there, incurring an added $1 billion in treatment charges. It is anticipated that stronger surveillance and control techniques now available can reduce incidence of these infections by 20 percent.

The United States has the most sophisticated infectious disease surveillance system in the world—and it is possible to target surveillance for many conditions—infectious and non-infectious—that are either preventable or amenable to effective intervention.

• • • •

In a broad prevention strategy, the concept of health protection must extend beyond traditional disease control measures to include protection against environmental and occupational hazards and reduction of accidental injuries.

These hazards are threats to all Americans, regardless of age, health status, or socioeconomic factors.

Yet many accidents can be prevented, toxic agents can be reduced, occupational safety and health programs can be implemented, community water supplies can be readily fluoridated, and infectious diseases can be effectively controlled and in some cases eliminated.

A commitment to safety and elimination of hazards—by everyone from government officials to parents to children—would save millions of Americans from needless pain and disability.

CHAPTER 10

HEALTH PROMOTION

Medical care begins with the sick and seeks to keep them alive, make them well, or minimize their disability.

Disease prevention begins with a threat to health—a disease or environmental hazard—and seeks to protect as many people as possible from the harmful consequences of that threat.

Health promotion begins with people who are basically healthy and seeks the development of community and individual measures which can help them to develop lifestyles that can maintain and enhance the state of well-being.

Clearly, the three are complementary, and any effective national health strategy must encompass and give due emphasis to all of them.

Beginning in early childhood and throughout life, each of us makes decisions affecting our health. They are made, for the most part, without regard to, or contact with, the health care system. Yet their cumulative impact has a greater effect on the length and quality of life than all the efforts of medical care combined.

Many factors increasing the risk of premature death can be reduced without medication. In fact, as we have noted, the striking decline in heart disease death rates in this country since the mid-1960s has coincided with reductions in several risk factors: cigarette smoking by men, consumption of high fat products, average serum cholesterol levels, and the number of people with untreated high blood pressure (Figure 10-A). During the same period in Europe, neither personal risk factors nor heart disease death rates declined.

Consider, too, the strikingly lower cancer rates among certain groups of Americans compared to those for the general population.

Seventh Day Adventists neither smoke nor drink, and about half follow a milk, egg and vegetable diet. For this group, not only is their cancer incidence, for those cancers strongly related to smoking and drinking, less than one seventh that of the general population; even their cancer incidence at other sites is only half to three-fourths as high. Similarly, Mormons, who also abstain from smoking and alcohol, have lower cancer rates.

And there are the promising results coming from recent efforts to organize community resources for health promotion.

Notable examples include the Stanford Heart Disease Prevention Program and the Multiple Risk Factor Intervention Trial (MRFIT), both funded by the National Heart, Lung, and Blood Institute.

The Stanford program, begun in 1972, has been monitoring the rates of cigarette smoking, serum cholesterol levels, and uncontrolled hyper-

FIGURE 10-A

PERCENT DECREASES IN RISK FACTORS FOR
CORONARY HEART DISEASE*

Risk Factor	Approximate Percent Decrease	Time Period
Cigarette smoking (% who smoke):		
Men	26	1964-1975
Women	8	
Per capita consumption of:		
Tobacco	22	1963-1975
Fluid milk and cream	20	
Butter	32	
Eggs	13	
Percent with high cholesterol (260 mg/100 ml plus):		
Men age 45-54	6	c1962-c1975
Men age 55-64	14	
Women age 45-54	13	
Women age 55-64	29	
Percent hypertensives untreated:		
In U.S.	10	c1962-c1974
In 14 U.S. cities†	25	

*Note: Coronary heart disease deaths (to which these risk factors are related) declined by 20 percent in the period 1968-1976.

†Part of a special National Heart, Lung, and Blood Institute study program.

tension in three Northern California communities. Two of the three employed active risk reduction activities, including messages designed for television, radio, newspapers and other media. In one of these two communities, face-to-face counseling also was provided for a sample of high risk individuals.

Within a two-year period in the two experimental communities, overall heart disease risk fell by about 25 percent. In both, there were reductions in average serum cholesterol and a six percent lowering of systolic blood pressures. A substantial reduction (net decrease of 35 percent) in smoking was achieved only among the high-risk individuals receiving counseling. In the community without an active information program, overall risk for heart disease actually increased during the first two years of the study.

The Multiple Risk Factor Intervention Trial program also seeks to change behaviors with respect to smoking, serum cholesterol, and high blood pressure. It is a multicenter clinical trial in 22 communities to determine whether, for men at high risk, a concentrated program based on counseling and directed simultaneously toward the three risks will result in a significant reduction in heart disease deaths.

Although final study results will not be available until 1983, preliminary data are especially encouraging with respect to the numbers of participants who have stopped smoking and those whose high blood pressure is under control. Moderate cholesterol reduction also has been achieved.

Abroad, promising results have come from a program in the province of North Karelia, Finland, which has the highest documented heart disease rate in the world.

In the early 70s, more than half of the men in North Karelia smoked; they also had extremely elevated cholesterol levels and high consumption of animal fats and dairy products; untreated hypertension was common.

Concerned about their high heart disease rate, North Karelians developed a massive health promotion campaign designed to help the 180,000 province residents control their blood pressure, reduce cholesterol intake, and stop smoking. Efforts included promotion of low-fat dairy products and low-fat sausages by local industries, training of local residents as health personnel, and extensive media coverage.

After five years there was an 18 percent drop in cigarette smoking among men ages 25 to 60 and a 15 percent decline among women. Butter consumption dropped and 50 percent of the population was using low-fat milk. The number of men with high blood pressure declined by 27 percent. Among women, the decline was 49 percent.

And significantly, preliminary results yet to be confirmed show a drop of 17 percent in heart attack incidence and 33 percent drop in the incidence of stroke among North Karelian men.

Here at home too, after the University of Southern California Medical Center ravamped its diabetic care system—by installing a telephone hotline for information and advice, making available counseling by physicians and nurses, and issuing pamphlets and posters to promote the service— emergency room visits per patient were halved and the incidence of diabetic coma decreased by two-thirds.

Relatively simple community health education programs, now increasing in number, can indeed make contributions.

This chapter deals with five types of behaviors which affect health and are targets for health promotion programs: smoking, alcohol and drug use, nutrition, exercise and fitness, and management of stress.

Smoking Cessation

Cigarette smoking is clearly the largest single preventable cause of illness and premature death in the United States.

It is associated, as Section II noted, with heart and blood vessel diseases; chronic bronchitis and emphysema; cancers of lung, larynx, pharynx, oral cavity, esophagus, pancreas, and urinary bladder; and with other ailments ranging from minor respiratory infections to stomach ulcers. Smoking during pregnancy also increases risks of complications of pregnancy and retardation of fetal growth.

Cigarette smokers have a 70 percent greater rate of death from all causes than nonsmokers, and tobacco is associated with an estimated

320,000 premature deaths a year. Another 10 million Americans currently suffer from debilitating chronic diseases caused by smoking.

A remarkable aspect of these statistics is that smoking presumably is voluntary, and theoretically all of this damage is therefore preventable.

Moreover, a large portion of a smoker's excess risk for heart disease disappears within two years after quitting—and within 10 to 15 years an exsmoker's chance of early death from a heart attack is no greater than that of someone who never smoked. If, in fact, all Americans stopped smoking, coronary deaths could be reduced by approximately 30 percent, with a saving of more than 200,000 lives a year. And people who have smoked for many years can reduce their risk of lung and urinary bladder cancer if they stop.

Changing Trends

In 1950, when the Nation first became generally aware of an association between smoking and lung cancer, there were about 18,000 lung cancer deaths. In 1964, the year of the first Surgeon General's Report on Smoking and Health, there were over 45,000 lung cancer deaths. An estimated 92,000 deaths from lung and related respiratory system cancers occurred in 1977.

The 1964 Surgeon General's Advisory Committee Report concluded that cigarette smoking was a cause of lung cancer in men and was associated with coronary artery disease, chronic bronchitis, and emphysema. Since then, cigarette smoking's relationship to these diseases—and to still others—has become clearer. A comprehensive review of the evidence linking smoking with a wide variety of health problems—with particular attention to special smoking-related problems for women, children and workers—is presented in the 1979 Surgeon General's Report on Smoking and Health.

The public's reaction to the risks of smoking can be measured by changes in cigarette consumption. In the early 1950s, consumption declined in response to the first scientific reports. It rose again, then dropped when the Surgeon General's Report was published in 1964, then rose a second time but dropped again between 1968 and 1970 as more television advertisements against smoking were aired.

All in all, more than 30 million smokers have quit since the first Surgeon General's Report, and the proportion of adult smokers has declined from about 42 percent in 1965 to a little more than one-third today. A large share of the decline is due to a drop in the proportion of men who smoke, but the percentage of women who smoke has decreased negligibly and there has been a doubling of the rate at which adolescent women (12 to 18 years) smoke.

Though the recent decline in the proportion of men who smoke is encouraging, an associated decline in cancer death rates may not appear for some years because cancer takes many years to develop. But the fall-off of heart disease deaths is undoubtedly due in part to the shift.

On the other hand, if the proportion of women who smoke does not decrease and current trends continue, experts predict that lung cancer will surpass breast cancer as the leading cause of cancer mortality among women by 1983.

Meanwhile, approximately 4,000 children and adolescents become cigarette smokers each day. While girls in the 1960s were smoking at about half the rate of boys, they now smoke as much. More than 20 percent of 12 to 17 year olds and about one-third of all 18 year olds now are regular smokers.

Approaches to the Problem

Much more can and must be done to educate the public about the risks of smoking.

Although Americans know about the relation between smoking and lung cancer, surveys show that they have yet to become aware that smoking-related cardiovascular diseases claim even more lives. And few believe they personally will suffer any harmful effects.

Physicians and dentists could be more helpful. Surveys show that only two-thirds of doctors and one-third of dentists routinely inquire about their patients' smoking habits. Only 25 percent of smokers say their physicians have told them to quit. Most physicians and dentists apparently wait until a serious smoking-related symptom or ailment has appeared, yet studies show that if doctors advise patients not to smoke, as many as 25 percent will quit or reduce the amount they smoke.

Most people say they intended to smoke for only a short time and well over half of new smokers confidently expect to stop within five years. The reality, however, is that once started the smoking habit is extremely difficult to overcome. About 90 percent of all current smokers have expressed a desire to quit.

To help smokers quit, many clinics, techniques, and devices have been developed over the past 20 years and different methods have succeeded to some extent with different individuals. But reverting back to smoking is a major problem for many people and effective techniques are needed to help exsmokers avoid tobacco.

Actually, 95 percent of smokers who successfully quit do so on their own. And four factors seem to be of major importance in their success: health concerns (including symptoms); a desire to set an example for others; a desire for self-control; and aesthetic reasons such as breath odor and loss of taste for food.

These motivations should therefore be stressed in anti-smoking literature, advertisements, and broadcast announcements, as well as in special information campaigns directed to such high risk groups as pregnant women, industrial workers in especially hazardous occupational settings, and persons with health problems likely to be worsened by smoking.

Special efforts should be directed to children and adolescents. School health education curricula are needed to help a child make intelligent decisions about smoking—as well as about other behavior affecting health—and to help reinforce those decisions against peer pressure and other forces that impel them toward serious risk-taking behavior.

Effective curricula already in existence need to be more widely used. Educational activities must begin at the earliest possible point in school and continue systematically throughout the child's educational experience.

The best of these programs emphasize not only knowledge of the human body but also how it works and how behavior affects it. They also impart attitudes of personal responsibility for protecting one's own health and means of coping with pressures and uncertainties.

Efforts for teenagers must be designed to help them deal with their own values and attitudes toward smoking and with their own sense of maturity. They should be aimed at helping them develop the ability to resist group pressures toward smoking and at reinforcing the concept that, in fact, smokers are the minority—not majority—both in their own age group and among adults.

One approach, which makes positive use of the peer pressures that influence youthful behavior, is deploying students themselves as health educators. Such peer instruction programs have shown substantial promise in preliminary trials.

Some have suggested use of economic sanctions such as increased taxes to discourage smoking. This is a complex political and economic issue not readily accomplished. But the effect of price changes—particularly of dramatic changes—on consumption merits further investigation.

Development of lower tar cigarettes has been urged as a means of reducing hazards. And smokers can take a first step toward quitting and hazard reduction by using low tar and nicotine cigarettes. They can also reduce hazards by not smoking to the end of a cigarette, by taking fewer puffs on each cigarette, by reducing inhalation and, gradually, the number smoked daily.

While gradual reduction is better than no reduction at all, it should be noted that generally smokers who quit all at once have better success than those who try to quit in steps.

Also, there is no known safe cigarette—including the low tar and nicotine varieties—nor any safe level of smoking for any type of cigarette. The smoker who continues to smoke, even in reduced amounts, still runs a significantly greater risk of illness and death than the nonsmoker.

Finally, the rights of nonsmokers should be recognized and supported. Measurable levels of nicotine have been found in the blood and urine of nonsmokers exposed to tobacco smoke. Such exposure may present a special health hazard for people with certain diseases. Breathing the smoke of others can lead to unsafe carbon monoxide levels, allergic reactions, and exacerbation of conditions such as asthma and bronchitis. For infants, risk of respiratory infections increases when parents smoke.

Legislation has been introduced in every state to restrict smoking in public places. Steps are being taken to restrict smoking in government buildings and facilities as well as on buses, airplanes, and passenger trains.

Despite all the difficulties, efforts to increase the number of nonsmokers should become much more energetic. The World Health Organization notes in a recent report: "The control of cigarette smoking could do more to improve health and prolong life in (developed) countries than any other single action in the whole field of preventive medicine."

Reducing Misuse of Alcohol and Drugs

Alcohol and other psychoactive substances exact a substantial toll of premature death, illness, and disability in the United States.

Alcohol

Because of its overuse and general social acceptance throughout American society, alcohol accounts for a significant share of the Nation's medical care cost burden.

Alcohol misuse is a factor in more than 10 percent of all deaths in the United States—about 200,000 a year. It is associated with half of all traffic deaths, many involving teenagers. Cirrhosis, which ranks among the 10 leading causes of death, is largely attributable to alcohol consumption. Alcohol use is also associated with cancer, particularly of the liver, esophagus and mouth. Primary liver cancer is almost exclusively attributed to alcohol consumption. People who drink and also smoke cigarettes have even greater increases in esophageal cancer rates. And excessive drinking during pregnancy can produce infants with severe abnormalities, including mental retardation.

Nor is the death and injury toll only for alcoholics or problem drinkers. Accidents, in particular, often involve the occasional drinker who is temporarily out of control.

Per capita consumption of alcohol by Americans increased during the 1960s—a trend generally attributed to the lowering of the legal drinking age in many States, an increase among young people consuming alcohol, and increasing use of alcohol by women.

The proportion of heavy drinkers in the population grew substantially in the 1960s to reach the highest recorded level since 1850, though it has leveled off in recent years. Drinking is greatest in the younger years and declines after age 50.

Currently, average consumption of alcohol for all persons older than 14 is 30 percent higher than 15 years ago—about 2.6 gallons of ethanol annually, representing a total of 28 gallons of beer, plus 2.5 gallons of distilled spirits and 2.25 gallons of wine.

Ten million adult Americans—seven percent of those 18 years or older—are estimated to be alcoholics or problem drinkers.

Of all adults who drink, more than a third have been classified as either current or potential problem drinkers, with women making up one-fourth to one-third of the latter. Youthful problem drinkers, aged 14 to 17 (intoxicated at least once a month) are estimated to number more than three million, between 20 and 25 percent of the age group.

The social and economic burdens associated with alcohol are enormous. Those who abuse drinking affect not only themselves but their 40 million family members as well. Alcohol abuse and alcoholism are estimated by the Alcohol, Drug Abuse and Mental Health Administration to have cost the Nation nearly $43 billion in 1975, including health and medical costs, lost production, motor vehicle accidents, violent crimes, fire losses, and social response programs.

Drugs

Although there is no question that drug misuse is a major problem, reliable information on actual prevalence is hard to obtain. Much depends on self-reporting and many problems occur among transient populations likely to be missed in any survey.

Moreover, interpretation of surveys is complicated by lack of agreement on what frequency of use of drugs constitutes abuse.

Heroin addiction, the most serious drug problem in the United States, appears to be declining. In 1978, there were an estimated 450,000 addicts, compared with an estimated 550,000 in 1975. It should be noted that the decline parallels demographic changes in the number of young adults.

The toll from highly addicting heroin includes premature death and severe disability, family disruption, and crime committed to maintain the habit. The heroin user is at very high risk of overdose death, of hepatitis and other infections from contaminated equipment and impurities in the drug, and from chronic undernutrition because money is spent on heroin instead of food. Preventing consequences of overdose and infection in users is virtually impossible since there is no control over the strength and purity of the drug or the means of administration.

Central nervous system depressants and stimulants with potential for abuse include many drugs ordinarily prescribed for their medical value. At least one million Americans are believed to misuse barbiturates or other sedative-hypnotic drugs and 30,000 are estimated to be addicted to them.

Excessive doses of depressants over a long period can result in both physical and psychological dependence, with abrupt withdrawal (particularly of barbiturates) leading to convulsions which may produce permanent disability or even death. Overdosing with barbiturates—intentional and accidental—is a leading cause of drug overdose fatalities but has declined somewhat as physicians have changed prescribing practices. Combinations of barbiturates with depressants, particularly alcohol, greatly increase the chance of death.

Cocaine is a stimulant which—despite its high cost—has become very popular for its propensity to induce euphoria and reduce feelings of fatigue. Some 10 million Americans have tried cocaine at least once and one to two million are current users. Although physical dependence does not develop, psychological dependence may. Some deaths due to toxic reactions to cocaine have been reported.

Hallucinogens, which distort perception of reality, can cause potentially fatal toxic reactions. And their unpredictable psychic effects may result in unintentionally dangerous behavior. One hallucinogen, PCP (phencyclidine hydrochloride), has a well-deserved street reputation as a "bad" drug, yet many people use it regularly, and in 1977 it was associated with at least 100 deaths and more than 4,000 emergency room visits.

Other illicit drugs—with less harmful physical and social consequences—are in more widespread use.

There are some 16 million current marijuana users. Among males 20 to 24 who have ever used marijuana, perhaps 17 percent are daily users. Among high school seniors recently surveyed, about 10 percent reported daily use. Of special concern is the relationship of marijuana to automobile accidents; especially when used in combination with alcohol, and by teenagers and young adults who are at high risk of accidents.

One of the dominant concerns about use of marijuana and other psychoactive drugs is the reduction in motivation and performance they may produce when used chronically, particularly by children and adolescents.

Prevention Programs

Helping people to stop or avoid starting misuse of alcohol or drugs will not be easy—particularly among population groups in which social and economic factors are prominent contributors to abuse of alcohol and drugs, and therefore complicate potential interventions.

For the broad range of alcohol and drug problems, strategies for intervention differ; but there are some common elements. They include: prevention through education that starts early and extends throughout life; altering the social climate of acceptability; reducing individual and social stress factors; and law enforcement.

One reason recent alcohol education efforts have had little success in changing children's behavior is that their moralistic nature has not always matched parental behavior or the favorable image afforded alcohol use in television advertising and programming. Such dichotomy creates confusion in young minds.

Similarly, efforts to educate young people about drug abuse dangers have met with skepticism—and, in fact, on occasion, the excitement and drama employed to discourage a drug's use have created an incentive to try the drug.

Educational strategies directed against drugs themselves appear to be less effective than those built around the concept of individual responsibility for the daily decisions that can affect health.

Young people who gain an understanding of how body systems work and how their personal choices affect their well-being are better prepared to make wise choices about alcohol and drug use. For this reason, comprehensive school health education programs directed toward strengthening children's decision-making capabilities may hold particular promise.

Moreover, because peer pressure, as noted earlier, has profound influence on youth behavior, educational programs that build on peer group counseling are more likely to be successful. School systems, youth-related organizations such as the Boys Club of America, Catholic Youth Organizations, 4-H and the Scouts, and churches and other community-based organizations can help develop such programs.

These programs serve many purposes. They open communication channels between adolescents and the health community; they teach young people tangible skills and give them important information, thus increasing their sense of self-worth; they also provide needed community services.

Our society needs to find more socially constructive outlets for the interests and energies of children and adolescents. While urbanization and farm mechanization have moved rapidly, alternative activities for the work once required have not been adequately developed. Challenging work for young people is important for more than economic reasons; it helps build self-respect and a better outlook for the future.

The media can be important in creating a social climate that encourages sound health-related personal decisions. In recent years, television has reduced its emphasis on the social acceptability of smoking—only, ironically, to have lighting a cigarette replaced in part by pouring a drink as a typical stage routine.

Labeling policies for alcohol and prescription drugs may provide an important means for conveying information which will help users to avoid harmful affects. Product labels may be especially useful for informing expectant mothers of the potential effects of ingested substances on the fetus.

Help and support must be offered to those already suffering from misuse problems. For alcohol-related problems, Alcoholics Anonymous, similar organizations for families of alcoholics, and workplace-based programs may be successful.

Health professionals need to play a more active role. A physician who diagnoses cirrhosis has no difficulty in recommending against alcohol use but may miss earlier opportunities to make the recommendation when the advice could make a difference.

Physicians and pharmacists can also be very important in reducing availability of legal drugs which may be abused. Physicians need to exercise more caution when prescribing psychoactive drugs, and pharmacists should check with physicians when in doubt about prescriptions.

Finally, legislation and law enforcement can help. The experience of some jurisdictions indicates that social practices may be substantially modified through vigorous enforcement of laws such as those against driving while intoxicated, and careful study of the efficacy of such measures is warranted.

Improved Nutrition

Although evidence keeps mounting that certain food factors and current dietary habits may be linked with health problems as diverse as heart disease, tooth decay, obesity and some types of cancer, consumers often find it difficult to make informed choices about food.

Most know that good nutrition can make a substantial contribution to health and development of infants and children and that healthy eating patterns should be firmly established in adolescents and young adults. Most also are aware that good nutrition is particularly important for pregnant women and the elderly.

But food choices are influenced by many complex factors and the consumer is often bombarded with an overload of somewhat confusing—and even conflicting—information from books, newspapers, magazine articles, and advertising.

Most diet deficiency diseases prevalent early in the century are now rarely seen. But iron deficiency in children and women of childbearing age remains a public health concern.

And although less than one percent of the American people can be considered undernourished in the traditional sense, data from the first Health and Nutrition Examination Survey by the National Center for Health Statistics show a trend toward low calorie intake among certain adults over age 45, and particularly among women over 60. If the trend continues, it is possible that some diet deficiency diseases may reappear.

Nevertheless, today's nutrition problems are still more likely to be associated with eating too much and with imbalance in the kinds of foods eaten than from eating too little.

The Obesity Problem

Thirty-five percent of women between ages 45 and 64 with incomes below poverty level and 29 percent of those with incomes above are considered obese, according to the National Center for Health Statistics. The comparable figures for men are five and 13 percent.

Obesity is clearly related to diabetes, gallbladder disease, and high blood pressure. In association with other risk factors, it can contribute significantly to heart disease. In addition to the physiological problems, obesity may have serious social consequences for the young person growing up in a society which prizes slimness and athletic ability.

A genetic component may be involved in some obesity. But the social environment of the family— eating and exercise habits and a tendency to view food as a "reward"—is of great importance. And, as noted in Chapter 4, obese children are three times more likely to be obese adults than children who are not overweight.

There is no quick, easy solution to obesity. Among adults, it has proved very difficult to reverse on a lasting basis.

Permanent weight loss has been found somewhat easier to achieve by people who inventory their food intake, avoid situations that would entice them to overeat, and gradually change their eating and exercise habits. Many nutritionally sound diets are available for weight control, but people should be extremely skeptical about fad diets promising rapid, painless weight reduction.

Obesity is not the only nutrition-related health problem. Cardiovascular disease and cancer are other public health concerns that may be dietrelated.

Nutrition and Cardiovascular Disease

A good case can be made for the role of high intake of cholesterol and saturated fat, usually of animal origin, in producing high blood cholesterol levels which are associated with atherosclerosis and cardiovascular diseases.

Animal studies have shown that reducing serum cholesterol can slow down and even reverse the atherosclerotic disease process.

And, in man, certain studies have shown: that people in countries where diets are low in saturated fats and cholesterol have lower average serum cholesterol levels and fewer heart attacks; and that Americans who habitually eat less fat-rich diets (vegetarians and Seventh-Day Adventists, for example) have less heart disease than other Americans. Other observations in man suggest the possibility that certain types of atherosclerosis may be reversed by cholesterol-lowering diets.

The weight of the evidence, therefore, now suggests that Americans who have been consuming high fat diets should attempt to reduce serum cholesterol by changing eating patterns. Moreover, these changes should begin at an early age. Not only adults but children in countries with low coronary heart disease rates have much lower serum cholesterol levels than many of our children have.

Many issues still need to be resolved. Among the most interesting are those concerned with high and low density lipoproteins (see Chapter 6). While it appears that a higher ratio of high-density to low-density lipoproteins carries a lower risk for heart disease, the effect of diet upon the ratio still is under study.

Some investigations indicate that the ratio is favorably influenced by lean body weight, regular vigorous exercise, smoking avoidance, consumption of small amounts of alcohol, and a diet with relatively more vegetables, fish and white meats than red meats. But further research is needed before definite statements can be made about diet and lipoproteins.

High dietary salt intake may produce high blood pressure, particularly in susceptible people. Unequivocally, studies in genetically predisposed animals show a cause-effect relationship between high salt intake and elevated blood pressure. Studies in man also suggest such a relationship and show, too, that when hypertension is present controlling salt intake can help combat it.

A prudent approach, given present knowledge, would be to limit salt consumption by cooking with only small amounts, refraining from adding salt to food at the table, and avoiding salty prepared foods. Careful label reading will reveal whether salt or a sodium compound has been added to a packaged food.

Diet and Cancer

The association between diet and cancer is more tenuous than between diet and heart disease.

Because populations with different dietary patterns have differing cancer rates—and emigrants assuming the patterns of their adopted country soon also assume new cancer rates—there has been much research into the possible diet-cancer association.

Studies in human populations have suggested a number of possibilities: that high consumption of animal protein may be linked to colon cancer; that low consumption of fiber from plant sources may also be linked to colon cancer; and that high consumption of fats, both saturated and unsaturated, may be linked to colon cancer and to hormone-related cancers of the ovary and prostate. All of these possibilities need further investigation.

Healthy Nutrition

Individual nutritional requirement variations make exact dietary standards impossible to establish. Variations also occur in the same person at different times—during pregnancy, with aging, during acute or chronic illness, or with changes in physical activity.

But given what is already known or strongly suspected about the relationship between diet and disease, Americans would probably be healthier, as a whole, if they consumed:

- only sufficient calories to meet body needs and maintain desirable weight (fewer calories if overweight);
- less saturated fat and cholesterol;
- less salt;
- less sugar;
- relatively more complex carbohydrates such as whole grains, cereals, fruits and vegetables; and
- relatively more fish, poultry, legumes (e.g., beans, peas, peanuts), and less red meat.

Adequate, balanced nutrition can be obtained by eating—in quantities sufficient to maintain desirable weight—a wide variety of foods each day, including meat or meat alternates, fruits and vegetables, cereal and bread-type products, and dairy products.

The processing of our food also makes a difference. The American food supply has changed so that more than half of our diet now consists of processed foods rather than fresh agricultural produce. Because of this change, we need more complete nutrient composition data about our food supply, particularly as related to some of the newer essential "trace minerals" such as molybdenum, manganese, chromium, and selenium.

The quantities of these trace minerals have not previously been a nutritional concern because practically everybody consumed a variety of fresh or minimally processed foods. Increased attention therefore also needs to be paid to the nutritional qualities of processed food.

Better Nutrition Education

Food choices are determined in part by the nutritional knowledge of the person who buys or prepares the food. Other factors include availability, personal and family likes and dislikes, and marketing and advertising practices. These factors should be addressed in educational initiatives to promote good food habits.

Until now, nutrition education has provided information rather than instruction in the skills that can be used to improve dietary habits.

Such skills should be taught in formal and informal nutrition education programs for people of all ages. And these programs should consider what too often has also been neglected in the past: the differences in food preferences found in different cultural groups.

Teachers, in particular, need to receive training in nutrition; and nutrition should be an integral part of the school curriculum.

More can also be done in medical care settings. Although education about nutritional intake is essential and often provided for patients suffering with health problems such as diabetes or kidney disease, it is uneven in quality.

And although pediatricians, obstetricians and other health workers often include some form of nutrition education as part of their care of infants, mothers, and pregnant women, rarely do they take advantage of this opportunity to build nutritional knowledge and positive attitudes for future decision-making.

Training in nutrition for physicians and other health professionals should have high priority, and nutrition training and services should be promoted in hospitals and clinics.

Sound nutrition information should also involve the media. Food advertising, particularly on television, has a powerful influence on food choices. Many foods are promoted for their convenience and ease of preparation or for their taste, rather than for nutritional value. Convenience and good taste are important considerations, but a balanced presentation should also consider nutritional value.

Results in the Stanford Heart Disease Prevention Program suggest that structured campaigns using multiple media sources can positively affect food selections to reduce, for example, consumption of products high in cholesterol or salt.

Education efforts must be augmented by direct food assistance to segments of the population finding it difficult to meet basic nutritional needs.

Certain older adults—for example, those with chronic diseases, acute illnesses, or particular genetic or lifestyle patterns—absorb nutrients less efficiently. But the primary problem for many of the elderly and other age groups is poverty and fixed incomes.

A number of Federal food distribution and supplemental food programs have been established to provide poor people with better diets. Among them are the nutrition services programs (including congregate and home-delivered meals), the Food Stamp Program, and the Special Supplemental Food Program for Women, Infants, and Children administered by the Department of Agriculture. Measures are needed to strengthen these programs and to assist people in using them.

Exercise and Fitness

For more than a generation, American living has become increasingly sedentary. Most of us drive or ride to work and most other places. Work itself, for much of the labor force, involves relatively little, if any, vigorous physical activity. Even in recreation, people commonly have tended to be spectators, not participants. The relative lack of physical activity has led to a decline in physical fitness among youth and adults alike.

Within the past half dozen years or so, however, there has been a promising resurgence of interest in physical exercise and fitness. A 1977 Gallup Poll found nearly half of American adults saying that they exercise regularly to keep fit. Millions participate in tennis, bicycling, swimming, calisthenics and other forms of exercise. Running, in particular, has become a very popular pastime even though it is in reality confined to a relatively small, and highly visible, portion of the population. (According to the National Center for Health Statistics, five percent of Americans over age 20, and 10 percent of men aged 20 to 44 run.)

Health Effects

Physical fitness activities affect health in many ways.

People who exercise regularly report that they feel better, have more energy, often require less sleep. Regular exercisers often lose excess weight as well as improve muscular strength and flexibility. Many also experience psychological benefits including enhanced self-esteem, greater self-reliance, decreased anxiety, and relief from mild depression.

Moreover, many adopt a more healthy lifestyle—abandoning smoking, excessive drinking, and poor nutritional habits.

Sustained exercise improves the efficiency of the heart and increases the amount of oxygen the body can process in a given period of time. Compared to non-exercisers, people who engage in regular physical activity have been observed to have one and a half to two times lower risk of developing cardiovascular disease, and an even lower risk of sudden death.

While not yet definitively proven, the role of exercise in preventing heart disease is attractive and plausible. An example of the growing evidence supporting the association between exercise and reduced cardiovascular risk comes from a study of 17,000 Harvard alumni. The physically active among them had significantly fewer heart attacks than the more sedentary. Those who expended less than 500 calories a week in exercise developed heart disease at about twice the rate of those expending 2,000 or more calories a week (approximately 100 calories are used for each mile run or walked). Regular, vigorous exercise was found to reduce risk of heart disease independently of other risk factors such as cigarette smoking or high blood pressure.

The kind of physical activity probably most beneficial to the cardiovascular system is sometimes called aerobic—exercise requiring large amounts of oxygen for energy production. Examples include brisk walking, climbing stairs, running, crosscountry skiing, and swimming.

An average of 15 minutes or more of aerobic exercise is thought to produce beneficial effects which are further increased when the exercise is done vigorously.

A reasonable goal for any individual ought to be 15 to 30 minutes of exercise at least three times a week. A beginner should start slowly and people over 40 should be examined by a physician first.

Non-aerobic activities, such as weight training and calisthenics, are useful for enhancing muscle tone, strength and flexibility. But they are often intermittent and less vigorous, and therefore may be less effective in reducing risk for cardiovascular disease.

The risk may be reduced by regular, sustained exercise in several ways. Such activity may cause the blood pressure of a hypertensive individual to fall an average of 10 points and may also lower serum cholesterol while raising the level of desirable high-density lipoproteins. It can also get rid of excess weight. Walking or running a mile daily—or swimming one-quarter mile—can lead to a reduction of more than 10 pounds in a year.

Aerobic exercise, when carefully prescribed, has been found useful for patients with chest pain (angina pectoris) and those recovering from heart attacks, enabling them to increase the amount of activity they can perform free of chest pain.

Such exercise has also been shown to be useful in treatment of other diseases. Asthmatics and people with chronic obstructive lung disease often can improve their respiratory capacity. Diabetics can lower their blood sugar levels and insulin requirements, and overweight adults who have become diabetic often are freed of any indications of the disease when they achieve normal weight through exercise and diet.

Gaps and Needs

Despite a doubling of the percentage of those who exercise, most participants do not exercise often or vigorously enough to achieve maximum health benefits.

Participation rates are higher among whites than minorities; among males than females; among younger than older persons; among the more educated than the less educated; among professionals than blue-collar workers; among the affluent than the poor; and among suburban-ites than city dwellers.

For children and adolescents, too often exercise involves an emphasis on team sports in which much of the time a player is inactive, and which are rarely engaged in later in life. More valuable would be prop-erly conducted physical education programs that could help promote lifetime habits of vigorous exercise as well as contribute to child growth and development.

Most older people do not exercise regularly. Yet suitable exercise programs can help them in many ways: by reversing the replacement of muscle by fat associated with inactivity; maintaining a good posture and muscular strength required for efficient movement in daily activities; improving joint mobility for the better balance skills needed for safety; and stimulating cardiorespiratory endurance.

Some people who exercise began on their own or because they were influenced by a friend. Other motivating influences include school, em-ployee health fitness programs, health professionals, media, and govern-ment programs.

In the early 1960s, responding to the emphasis by President John F. Kennedy through his Council on Youth Fitness, many schools under-took more extensive fitness programs and a number of States began to require daily physical education for school children.

But since the late 1960s, many school physical education programs have had to cut back for lack of adequate State and local funding. Many States today have only limited requirements for physical educa-tion and no requirements at all for some grade levels. It has become even more important for parents to see that their children are exercising adequately.

During the past few years, an increasing number of employee fitness programs have been developed in business and government. Some com-panies have full-time fitness directors in charge of programs. In the most successful activities, participation rates range up to 40 percent, with benefits accruing to management as well as to workers who, feeling better, often may work better.

Health professionals have largely ignored active promotion of suitable exercise for their patients. A recent survey found 80 percent of patients not remembering that their physicians had ever recommended exercise. When exercise was recommended, it was usually of nonvigorous nature with limited value. More interest and concern by health professionals could do much to get more people exercising.

On a national level, government involvement has largely been through the President's Council on Physical Fitness and Sports. Since 1956, the Council has provided impressive leadership in drawing attention to the importance of exercise and fitness. It has assisted in development of employee health programs, public information programs, and special projects designed to increase participation in fitness and sports activities.

But what is needed is a substantial national effort involving all levels of both public and private sectors.

Stress Control

Stress is normal, inevitable; a part of life. It is experienced in family relationships, school, work, traffic, shopping, financial and other problems. And everyone develops means of coping—more or less effectively.

Some means of coping are beneficial—as, for example, when the response is an effort to improve performance.

But there are destructive responses such as excessive alcohol use, resorting to drugs, violence, reckless behavior, depression, and other forms of mental illness.

There are indications that stress can be related to cardiovascular disease and deaths, gastrointestinal disorders, and other diseases and physical health problems as well as much mental illness.

Studies have indicated that stress in the home, for example, can increase a child's risk of streptococcal throat infection—and an expectant mother's risk of pregnancy complications.

One revealing study assessed pregnant women, married, of similar age, race, and social status, all of whose babies were delivered in the same hospital. The finding: those women undergoing a great deal of social stress and lacking strong social supports—measured by closeness of ties with husband, family, and community—had almost three times the frequency of complications of pregnancy or delivery.

People under stress experience measurable changes in body functions: a rise in blood pressure and secretion of adrenaline and other hormones at higher levels. The changes are basically defensive, mobilizing body energies to meet a threat.

But when stress—or an individual's reaction to it—is excessive, physiologic changes can be so dramatic as to have serious physical and emotional consequences.

135

Reducing the Harmful Consequences of Stress

Two strategies are needed to minimize destructive stress consequences: preventing or reducing stress itself and improving individual stress-coping skills.

Opportunities for stress prevention exist in the work setting. Many jobs are dull, boring, or dangerous. Many people work under unpleasant circumstances—noise, polluted air, cramped quarters. The fear of losing one's job is an important source of stress.

Many of these factors, as noted earlier, can be eliminated or reduced. The work environment can be improved. Job assignments can be better tailored to individual interests and capabilities. Such improvements may pay dividends in increased productivity and decreased absenteeism and job turnover rates as well as reduced stress for the individual workers.

In the community setting, stress for individuals and groups often can be reduced through helping networks, neighborhoods, and community organizations.

The recent report of the President's Commission on Mental Health noted the significance of support systems in fostering a sense of security and as an effective treatment measure for people suffering problems associated with both physical and mental health.

There is extensive evidence of the importance of a sense of neighborhood or belonging for people and of the meaningful roles in people's lives played by neighborhood institutions such as churches, schools, ethnic clubs, fraternal organizations, community organizations, and others.

In a pluralistic society, people meet needs and solve problems in varied ways. And a neighborhood-based approach—with community support systems designed to address diverse individual needs—can be critical to individual well-being.

Strengthening neighborhood networks can help people in many ways: to gain a sense of control over their lives; reduce alienation from society; improve capacity to solve new problems; and maintain the motivation to overcome handicaps or the frustrations common in modern society.

With adequate day care programs, for example, stressful pressures on working mothers can be reduced. The stressful consequences of unwanted teenage pregnancy and motherhood can be substantially reduced by programs that enable the young women to complete their educations and qualify for satisfactory employment.

Racial and ethnic tensions can be eased through community action to improve cooperation and understanding. Young people at highest risk of becoming school dropouts can be identified and programs can be designed to anticipate and help meet their needs. Elderly people in need of support after retirement or loss of a spouse can be identified and helped through community services.

Efforts to improve coping skills must begin with an understanding of the events most difficult to handle emotionally.

Extensive research in this area has generally confirmed folk wisdom. The death of a spouse, the serious illness of a child, the loss of a job, family disruption and divorce, and other catastrophic changes over which the individual has little or no control, are the stresses most likely to cause psychosomatic disorders or other emotional problems, and their consequences.

Since stressful events are not always preventable, preparation for dealing with them needs to begin early. Emphasis should be given to building coping skills in children and young people. Too often, stress has been addressed only after the problem is fully developed—by treatment of the alcoholic, the drug abuser, the acutely depressed person, and by penalties for criminal offenders. Much more attention should be given to preparing people to deal in less destructive ways with unavoidable stresses.

To help young people and adults deal with critical stresses as they arise, a number of self-help and mutual support activities have been developed in communities across the country. Many evolved from the crisis intervention centers of the late 1960s. They deal with a wide range of stress-generated or stress-related problems: alcoholism, pregnancy, divorce, suicide attempts, rape, terminal illness, death of a child, death of a spouse, and many others.

There are in addition self-help, mutual aid groups for the handicapped; drug abusers; parents of handicapped children; parents who abuse their children; young people in search of jobs and identity; widows; old people; patients who have heart attacks, colostomies or mastectomies; gamblers; smokers; drinkers; overeaters; and many more. These groups constitute a significant community resource.

Although the group programs may vary in effectiveness, their rapid spread indicates they may be responding to social needs not completely filled by families, churches, schools, or health and mental health professionals.

Helping to prevent suicide is a particularly important task.

Health professionals who see people at high risk—and the families and friends of such people— may be able to assist by carefully assessing their emotional status and providing, or referring them to, appropriate help.

Guns, alcohol, barbiturates and other drugs with lethal potential are used in a large proportion of suicide attempts. Their availability and use could be controlled more effectively.

Suicide also can be prevented by indirect means. Notably, in England, when the carbon monoxide content of gas piped to homes was reduced, suicides as well as accidental deaths dropped sharply. And while what had been the most common means of committing suicide was virtually eliminated, there was no compensating increase in suicide by other means.

A vital part of community strategy to reduce harmful stress consequences is to assure that people know about available services—and that services are truly accessible in terms of location and hours of operation. This applies to hotlines and sources of professional counseling as well as self-help and other supportive services.

For this, local media, telephone directories, churches, civic organizations, and other outreach channels can be used.

And there must be an effort to have services offered in ways that assure that no stigma attaches to their use.

Not least of all, there should be educational efforts by health professionals, schools, and all community groups and services to underscore the importance of the family as a potential resource for individuals trying to cope with stressful situations. How families develop communications between parents and children, offer support to a troubled member, and care for needs and views of family elders can either trigger or intensify stress on the one hand, or, on the other, help significantly to ameliorate it.

To be sure, stress is inevitable with living. But excessively stressful factors in the environment can be assessed; many can be reduced or removed; and families and educational, social service, and other support programs can help people cope effectively with those that remain.

Exactly how much can be achieved by strong, multi-faceted community programs to deal with stress is difficult to predict. But certainly it is important to test the extent to which such programs can reduce the individually and socially devastating effects of failure to cope adequately: homicides, suicides, substance abuse, accidental deaths and injuries, and disease.

Even relatively minor reductions would amply repay the investment.

• • • •

Collectively, smoking, misuse of alcohol and other drugs, poor dietary habits, lack of regular exercise, and stress place enormous burdens on the health and well-being of many Americans today.

Identifying and implementing ways to help people adopt more healthful habits will require a large commitment from government, schools, media, health professionals, and business and industry.

It will be necessary, too, to work to reduce pressures in our society which often lead people to adopt unhealthy habits.

Although helping people to understand the need for and to act to change detrimental lifestyles cannot be easy, the dramatic potential benefits clearly make the effort worthwhile.

SECTION IV
CHALLENGE TO THE NATION

CHAPTER 11

CHALLENGE TO THE NATION

Americans are becoming healthier people—but more can be achieved.

This report has described and documented the potential for better health at each stage of life. It has set forth specific goals to be attained over the next decade, and a full agenda of possible actions to be taken.

To reach these goals will require a national effort and the commitment of people extending far beyond what we traditionally consider the health sector. No single segment of society can accomplish them alone. Unnecessary death and disability can be prevented—and better health can be maintained—only through a partnership that involves the serious commitment of individual citizens, the communities in which they live, the employers for whom they work, voluntary agencies, and health professionals.

Government agencies at all levels must encourage and bolster their efforts.

How to move expeditiously toward the goals of prevention is the challenge for the years to come.

The Obstacles

Expectations for programs in disease prevention and health promotion must be geared to realities. Social factors, personal attitudes, economics, and the knowledge base all are potential restraints to progress.

Socioeconomic factors. The critical influence of adequate income, housing, diet, education, and healthful workplaces in shaping the health of our people deserves continuing and serious attention. Without adequate resources to solve problems in these areas, the health of vulnerable population groups is at risk.

The Director General of the World Health Organization has said that economic development and health are indivisible. This holds true for the disadvantaged in our population.

Fundamental social and economic improvement is essential to better health for Americans.

Personal attitudes. Formidable obstacles also exist on other fronts. Prominent among them are individual attitudes toward the changes necessary for better health. Though opinion polls note greater interest in healthier lifestyles, many people remain apathetic and unmotivated.

Illness is often still viewed as a matter of random chance, not to be averted but to be tolerated and accepted.

Some consider activities to promote health moralistic rather than scientific; still others are wary of measures which they feel may infringe on personal liberties.

However, the scientific basis for suggested measures has grown so compelling, it is likely that such biases will begin to shift.

Economics. Resistance may also be expected from certain industries. The threat of economic loss due to decreased use of a product, or to requirements for sometimes costly measures to protect workers and the public, can lead to vigorous opposition to efforts to promote health or prevent disease and disability.

Knowledge. The knowledge base for prevention activities is growing dramatically, but there is still a need to learn more. Better measures are needed to: further identify causes of diseases; detect and test potential hazards; provide people with information which will motivate them and provide them with the skills to control behaviors they are trying to change.

More accurate techniques must be developed with which to estimate program costs and measure program effectiveness.

Opportunities for Action

We cannot afford to wait for perfect solutions before beginning to act. Many specific measures are available and must be taken to facilitate opportunities for better health.

Appendix I summarizes the measures which can be taken to enhance our prospects for better health at the major life stages. Responsibility for facilitating these actions falls to people at many levels.

Individuals. Each of us has a tremendously important role, as noted throughout this report. Personal lifestyles are responsible for a large share of unnecessary disease and disability in the United States.

People decide day by day and hour by hour what foods to eat, how much to consume, whether or not to smoke a cigarette or take a drink of alcohol. Greater or lesser amounts of physical activity are chosen. Various ways of coping with stress are developed.

Important decisions are also made about what services to seek, what conditions to be screened for.

People can determine not only what services to use, but the nature of those services as well. Individual participation in community decisions can affect the availability of health services, the quality of the environment, and other issues with health implications.

Each of these decisions influences the length of people's lives and their capacity to enjoy it.

Families. An individual's responsibility extends to others as a parent, a marriage partner, and a neighbor. One person's choice in health behavior can affect the choices of others.

The role as exemplar and guide is particularly critical for the parent who is shaping the health practices of another generation. Parents can enhance the opportunities for their children's health by fostering healthy personal habits, by ensuring availability and use of appropriate childhood health services, by participating in sound and enjoyable recreational activities, and by encouraging the development of effective health curricula in the school systems.

Health professionals. Physicians, nurses, and other health professionals have a particular opportunity and obligation to provide information and services necessary to promote better health and prevent disease.

People continue to note that they would be more likely to try to change their behaviors if their physicians strongly recommended such changes. Yet health professionals often find themselves too pressed by duties related to diagnosis and treatment to capture the opportunity they have to influence the behavior, and therefore the health, of their patients.

These professionals need to be trained to view themselves as educators and models, as well as practitioners of a particular discipline.

Health institutions. Hospitals and other health institutions, likewise, need not only be concerned with the sick.

Some hospitals are now actively providing preventive services and organizing community health promotion efforts. Some Health Maintenance Organizations, structured with incentives to keep their members healthy, have also helped expand preventive services.

Other incentives to good health can be provided by insurance companies through offering preferential rates on life and health insurance to groups engaged in health promotion programs at the worksite.

Schools. More than 40 million children and youth spend most of their day in school. No group is more able than school teachers to provide information and instruction that can help young people make decisions that promote good health.

Comprehensive school health education activities can: enhance a child's skills and personal decision-making; promote understanding of the concepts of health and the causes of disease; and foster knowledge about the ways in which one's health is affected by personal decisions related to smoking, alcohol and drug use, diet, exercise, and sexual activity.

Business and labor. Business leaders, working with their labor counterparts, can make substantial contributions to health through programs and services provided for employees, and through responsible manufacturing and marketing practices which embrace health concerns.

The worksite may provide an appropriate setting for health promotion as well as health protection activities. A number of companies have already shown leadership in providing employee fitness programs and encouraging worker participation, but more can be done.

Furthermore, business practices in advertising products may play a key role in influencing consumer behavior.

To date, the net effect in many areas of advertising—particularly for food products, over-the-counter drugs, tobacco, and alcohol—has generally not been supportive of health promotion objectives. But, as some companies are now recognizing, in an increasingly health conscious climate health promotion can result in excellent corporate public relations, as well as save money, through programs to improve the health of their own employees.

Communities. Most communities have substantial resources, sometimes unrecognized, for prevention and health promotion.

Included in these resources are the networks of voluntary agencies, media broadcasters, and civic and religious programs. All can provide a variety of useful services and help to create a climate of interest in better health.

Certainly the voluntary organizations have played the major role to date in drawing people's attention to important health issues.

Public forums provided by media sources, such as television, radio, newspapers, and magazines, and by commercial enterprises such as grocery and department stores, can also be used creatively to facilitate the deployment of health promotion and disease prevention measures.

Government. The American system for delivering health care services is pluralistic, and government at all levels—Federal, State, and local—operates direct care services for many beneficiary groups.

Federal facilities provide care to veterans, American Indians, the armed forces, merchant seamen, and others. State and local governments operate systems serving the mentally ill, the disadvantaged, and other groups. Through grants and contracts, government helps to support health care delivered through a still greater variety of agencies. Finally, through such programs as Medicare and Medicaid, government helps pay the bills for health care delivered in virtually every facility in the United States.

All provide potential means to deliver preventive services.

Federal and State governments have other important responsibilities in disease prevention and health promotion: to provide leadership in setting priorities and goals for prevention activities; to help expand the knowledge base through research and data collection; to assure that preventive services are provided to high risk groups on a priority basis; to determine and enforce health and safety standards protecting people; and, if necessary, to provide economic incentives to encourage health and safety.

The importance of local governmental units to successful prevention programs is unquestioned. The past successes of prevention and public health have been predominantly community based.

Local sanitation measures, purification of community water supplies, surveillance and control of epidemics have all been community matters. More recently, fluoridation of community water supplies has been the greatest single measure promoting dental health, though many communities lack its benefits.

Local government, assisted and supported by its State and Federal counterparts, can establish and enforce important regulations—rodent control, housing codes which address such problems as lead-based paint, air and water pollution control, and laws requiring immunization as a prerequisite to attending school.

• • • •

The diversity of participants in prevention activities is both necessary and desirable. What has been lacking up to now, however, has been a mechanism for coordinating these various efforts and bringing focus and direction to new ones to fill gaps.

Responsibility for implementing the newer approaches to health promotion and disease prevention has for the most part rested everywhere, and thus nowhere.

However, opportunities may be emerging to link and coordinate the resources available at various levels. Many governors, county officials, and mayors are in the process of developing mechanisms to meet new needs in prevention.

Furthermore, the 205 newly-created health systems agencies and State health planning bodies provide a potential means of fostering the actions outlined in this report to respond to the needs and characteristics of their respective populations.

What is most apparent is that the effort must be truly a collective one. While the measures are readily within our capabilities, their realization will require diligence, determination, and cooperation.

If the commitment is made at every level, we ought to attain the goals established in this report, and Americans who might otherwise have suffered disease and disability will instead be healthy people.

APPENDIXES

APPENDIX I

MEASURES FOR BETTER HEALTH: A SUMMARY

Throughout this report a number of specific measures have been identified as important to improving the health of individuals. Summarized in this Appendix are the principal recommendations for healthier infants, children, adolescents and young adults, adults and older adults.

In most cases, issues which span several age groups are discussed for the age group at greatest risk for the problem addressed. However, for those issues in which the nature of the problem varies by life stage (e.g., nutrition), the recommendation is repeated with a different emphasis for each age group.

HEALTHY INFANTS

Education for parenthood. People who are well informed about the care required by infants can better plan and prepare for parenthood. Prospective parents can seek education-for-parenthood classes through physicians, hospitals, and community organizations. Schools can offer preparation for parenthood to children and teenagers.

Genetic counseling. Prospective parents who have a history of family disorders such as Down syndrome, Tay-Sachs disease, sickle cell anemia, hemophilia, muscular dystrophy, or serious mental disorders should seek special counseling. Health professionals can provide this information to their patients and make appropriate referrals for genetic services.

Prenatal care. Good prenatal care is essential for a healthy pregnancy. Medical care, dietary assistance and counseling are important for all expectant mothers. Mothers with social and economic barriers to such care can be targeted by outreach and follow-up programs.

Prenatal nutrition. Pregnant women have extra needs for iron, protein, calcium, and calories and may need to be provided with dietary suggestions and/or supplements. Nutritional guidance and services are available from health professionals and service agencies.

Prenatal maternal habits. To reduce the potential for adverse effects on the developing fetus, women should avoid tobacco and alcohol during pregnancy. Counseling and appropriate services can help expectant mothers who wish to avoid these risks. Similarly, physicians should avoid prescribing use of medications and exposure to radiation by pregnant women, unless warranted by special circumstances.

Amniocentesis. A test (amniocentesis) sampling the intrauterine fluid at about the 16th week of pregnancy can determine whether certain serious birth defects exist in the fetus. Expectant mothers at higher risk include those who: are 35 and over; have a history of multiple spontaneous abortions; or have a family history of Down syndrome, neural tube defects, inherited metabolic disorders, multiple birth defects, or sex-linked inherited disorders. Detection of an abnormality may require a personal decision about an abortion.

Breast feeding. Breast milk is the most complete form of infant nutrition and is recommended for full-term newborn babies, unless there are specific problems or breast feeding is unsuccessful. If a nursing mother is healthy and well nourished, fluoride and possibly Vitamin D may be the only supplements needed by the baby. After about four months iron may also have to be added. Solid foods should not be introduced hastily into the baby's diet—rather they should be phased in gradually.

Pediatric care. Regular, comprehensive pediatric care can help assure the early detection of preventable problems, and provide preventive services such as immunizations (see below). In addition to a detailed examination after birth, every baby should be examined before leaving the hospital or within 10 days of birth, and again at approximately two, four, six, and nine months of age.

Immunizations. Childhood diseases that can be prevented by vaccinations continue to be a threat to infant health. Babies should be immunized for diphtheria, pertussis, tetanus, and polio at ages two months, four months, and six months (polio immunization is optional at six months). They should also receive the recommended childhood immunizations thereafter.

Social services. Some families require special support services to enhance the healthy growth and development of their children. Such services include high quality day care, improved foster care and adoption programs, as well as services to assist families in which a parent may suffer from chronic disabling disease, mental illness, alcoholism, or drug abuse.

HEALTHY CHILDREN

Early childhood development. A stimulating and healthy environment during the early part of life can enhance a child's growth and development. Programs such as Head Start, which provide comprehensive services for children, including day care, health care, nutrition, education and counseling, have produced important gains in child development, particularly for families with low incomes.

Special support services. Special sources of support should be available through community agencies and health care providers to assist children and families under particular stress. Foster care programs and practices should be designed to increase the opportunities for children to grow up in a stable and healthy environment.

Injury reduction. Accidents are the single greatest threat to children's health. People can reduce children's risk of injury and death by:
  • having the child secured in an approved child carrier, safety harness or seat belt when riding in an automobile;

- storing toxic agents out of reach, away from food, and in special containers with fastened safety caps;
- ensuring against access to knives and guns;
- carefully supervising young children at play, particularly when they are near water or streets;
- instructing the child what to do in situations of special risk (e.g., stoves, matches, electrical sockets, traffic).

Pediatric care. Some childhood problems can be prevented or ameliorated through the provision of certain medical sevices. Examples of such services include: identification and treatment of vision and hearing problems; assessment of developmental skills important to learning; immunizations (see below); and early diagnosis and treatment of childhood infections. Children should, therefore, receive routine pediatric evaluations at least every two to three years.

Immunizations. Children should be immunized for diphtheria, pertussis, tetanus, and polio at ages two months, four months, six months, 18 months, and four to six years (polio immunization is optional at six months), and for measles, mumps, and rubella at age 15 months.

Nutrition and exercise. Acquiring healthy eating and exercise habits in childhood may have lifelong benefits. An appropriate balance of food intake and physical activity promotes normal weight. Excessive intake of salt, sugar, and fats should be avoided. Parents and schools can emphasize these points through instruction, meal planning, and physical education programs emphasizing lifelong exercise activities. Nutrition supplements can be provided to children in high risk families.

Healthy habits. Preparing young children for peer group pressures with regard to smoking, alcohol use, drug use, and sexual activity can enhance their ability to deal with those pressures later. Parents, schools, and health professionals are all important to the provision of comprehensive health education which can help children to acquire skills to cope with problems they will confront as teenagers.

Fluoridation. The most effective and efficient way to prevent tooth decay is through fluoridation of community water supplies. If the water supply is not fluoridated, alternative fluoride sources can be provided through school-based fluoride mouth rinse or tablet programs, fluoride rinsing services from dentists, and fluoride tablets for home use.

Dental care. Children should be taught proper tooth brushing and flossing techniques at early ages, and should begin regular visits to a dentist by age three. Sweets in the diet should be limited to prevent tooth decay.

HEALTHY ADOLESCENTS AND YOUNG ADULTS

Roadway safety. Autombile accidents are the leading cause of death among young people. A substantial number of injuries and deaths could be avoided through careful, defensive driving habits. Especially important are: avoiding driving after drinking (or riding with a driver who has been drinking) or use of mood-altering drugs; obeying traffic laws; and using seat belts or, for cyclists, helmets. These efforts can be reinforced by Federal, State, and local measures to set and enforce safety regulations and lower speed limits, and to improve roadway and vehicular design.

Smoking, alcohol, and drug use. Experimental behavior by young people can lead to dependence or misuse of certain substances. Collective measures can be taken by parents, teachers, health professionals, and community organizations to provide adolescents and young adults with information and skills necessary to help them avoid cigarette smoking or harmful use of alcohol or drugs.

Nutrition and exercise. Changes in values and social pressures may encourage adolescents to eat snack foods that do not contain adequate supplies of essential nutrients. Yet, good eating habits and regular, vigorous exercise are important to still growing adolescents. During their growth spurt, teenagers need more calories, and particularly more protein, calcium, and iron.

Family planning. Unwanted pregnancy is a distressing problem for adolescent and young adult women in this country. Families, schools, health professionals, and social organizations can ensure that information about birth control measures is provided to young people of both sexes, and that family planning services are easily accessible to those who are sexually active. Services (including continued schooling) can also be made available in the community for young women who become pregnant and are in need of care and advice.

Sexually transmissible diseases. Sexually transmissible diseases that affect large numbers of young people are preventable. Families, schools, health professionals and social organizations can help provide information, confidential counseling, and treatment to prevent the transmission of venereal diseases. Periodic screening for disease which may not be symptomatic can be obtained from private physicians and community clinics, and encouraged for sexually active young people. Clinic personnel, sex educators, and family planning services counselors can stress the value of condoms in reducing the spread of disease and can emphasize the importance of informing partners immediately if disease is discovered.

Immunization. Young people should receive a booster immunization for diphtheria and tetanus at age 15.

Mental health. Young people frequently experience periods of frustration, uncertainty, and confusion, and should be encouraged to talk over problems with people with whom they can be open. Alert and sensitive friends, family members, clergy, or counselors at school or work can be helpful during periods of stress, anxiety, depression or uncertainty. Hotlines may also be helpful. Mental health professionals may be needed if conditions persist.

Firearms. Handguns are involved in a substantial number of homicides, suicides and accidental deaths in this country. Actions at the individual, community, and governmental levels can provide measures to reduce the availability of handguns.

HEALTHY ADULTS

Smoking. Cigarette smoking is the principal preventable cause of chronic disease and death in this country. Public education efforts at the Federal, State, and local levels, as well as health professionals, can provide information about the health hazards of smoking and suggestions on how to stop. Those who cannot quit on their own may benefit from one of the organized smoking cessation clinics. Those who are unable or unwilling to stop ought to smoke brands low in tar and nicotine, to inhale less, to smoke their cigarettes only half way, and to reduce gradually the number of cigarettes smoked.

Alcohol. Misuse of alcohol leads to accidental injury, family disruption, and chronic disease for millions of Americans. It is important that people realize the dangers—particularly for pregnant women—when alcohol is used excessively. Individuals (or their families) with alcohol-related problems may find effective assistance from health professionals, the clergy, community groups such as Alcoholics Anonymous, or programs run by various businesses to assist employees with drinking problems.

Nutrition. Good nutrition is an essential component of good health. People should adopt prudent dietary habits, consuming:
- only sufficient calories to meet body needs (fewer calories if the person is overweight);
- less saturated fat and cholesterol;
- less salt;
- less sugar;
- relatively more complex carbohydrates, such as whole grains, cereals, fruits and vegetables; and
- relatively more fish, poultry, legumes (e.g., peas, beans, peanuts), and less red meat.

Employers, food advertisers, grocery stores, and health and social service agencies can add to the promotion of healthy nutritional habits by providing the information and access to foods necessary to a good diet.

Exercise. Regular exercise can bring physical and psychological benefits. Adults should be encouraged to exercise vigorously—if possible, at least three times a week for about 15 to 30 minutes each time. Caution should, however, be taken to initiate activity gradually, and anyone over 40, or with a health problem of any kind, should consult a physician before beginning a vigorous exercise program. The importance of regular and sustained exercise for adults should be stressed in public information programs and by health professionals. Communities and employers can encourage fitnessrelated programs, including, where practical, the provision of facilities or pathways to make bicycling, running, and other exercise safer and more convenient.

Environmental health. Toxic agents in our environment can present health hazards which may not be detected for years. Private and public actions at all levels are important to protect against possible environmental hazards. Individuals can support the monitoring of industrial and agricultural production processes to reduce exposure to potentially toxic agents.

Worksite health and safety. The occupational setting is important both as a source of potential health hazards and a site for health promotion activities. Health programs at the worksite can provide information and protection related to all potential workplace hazards for employees, including stress, as well as offer activities and services to promote healthier lifestyles. People should both encourage these programs and take advantage of them.

Hypertension. High blood pressure affects millions of Americans and is a major contributor to heart disease and stroke. Adults should have a screening exam for high blood pressure at least every five years, and every two to three years if over age 40. If hypertension is discovered, and medication prescribed, it is important that people follow their therapeutic regimens carefully.

Pap smear. The Pap smear is an important tool to detect cervical cancer at early stages. Women should have three Pap smears taken one year apart beginning at age 20, or at the beginning of sexual activity. Thereafter, a Pap smear should be taken every three years. Screening frequency should be increased if any abnormalities are found, or if a woman is taking oral contraceptives or estrogen therapy.

Breast examination. Self-examination is the most effective way to detect breast cancer at an early treatable stage. Women should examine their own breasts monthly, after the menstrual period, for early signs of cancer (lumps, abnormal discharge, irregular size). Post-menopausal women should select a specific day of the month for such self-examination. Health professionals and public health education programs can provide information and instruction on breast self-examination, and increase their efforts to disseminate this important information. Periodic screening by mammography is not needed until after age 50, except for women who have already had cancer in one breast, and after 40 for women with a family history of breast cancer.

Cancer signs. Some cancers present signs at early stages in which the chances for successful treatment are greater. People should watch for early signs of cancer and consult a physician if any are noticed. In addition to the signs for breast cancer noted above, other cancer signs include: changes in bowel or bladder habits; a sore that does not heal; unusual bleeding or discharge; difficulty swallowing; change in a wart or mole; or nagging cough or hoarseness (American Cancer Society's seven cancer signs).

Mental health. Many people suffer from various forms of emotional disorders or mental illness. It is quite common for people to become, at one time or another, uncommonly anxious, depressed, or have difficulty coping with a life event. Professional assistance may be helpful if particular difficulty is encountered and may be available through health professionals, employers, local media, community organizations, hospitals, telephone hotlines, and other outreach organizations.

Dental care. People frequently lose their teeth prematurely because of poor dental and gum care. Adults should take care of their teeth with daily brushing and flossing and an annual dental examination.

HEALTHY OLDER ADULTS

Work and social activity. Employment and/or volunteer opportunities are important for older people accustomed to working. Maintaining an active social life is also important to their good health. Older people should remain active socially, avoid isolation, and maintain ties with family members and friends. Community health and social organizations can facilitate group activities for older people, when possible, in community centers.

Exercise. Regular physical activity for older adults can provide physical and psychological benefits, as well as help maintain flexibility and balance important to preventing falls. Older adults should therefore engage in exercise, such as daily walks, regularly.

Nutrition. Older people have certain special dietary needs. Regular, nutritious meals are important and particular care should be taken to include vegetables, sources of iron, calcium, and fiber, and use more fish, poultry, and legumes than red meat as sources of protein in the diet.

Preventive services. Some problems associated with aging can be detected and corrected at early stages. Older adults should have health check-ups at least every two years until age 75, and every year thereafter. The following should be performed each time: blood pressure check (with follow-up and treatment, if warranted), hearing and vision exam, breast exam for women, urinalysis, and hematocrit (measurement of red blood cells). At less frequent intervals women should have Pap smears, and all should have stool examined for blood. When possible, these and other preventive services such as foot care, dental care and dietary guidance should be provided at a single location.

Medication. Older people frequently receive too much medication. Often, fewer kinds of medications and lower dosages will suffice. Patients should ask their physicians to regularly review the medications they are taking. They should also request that medication be prescribed by its generic name, whenever feasible.

Immunization. Every year, many older adults die or are incapacitated unnecessarily due to influenza or pneumonia. Older people can consult their physicians about immunization against these diseases.

Home safety. Falls are the leading cause of accidental injury and death among older adults. People and agencies responsible for housing for the elderly can provide such home safety measures as ample lighting, sturdy railings and steps, non-slip floor surfaces, and fire protection and detection measures.

Services to maintain independence. For those whose activity is limited, often relatively minor services can help older people maintain their independence. People should encourage programs and services to help avoid unnecessary institutionalization. Examples include programs for: safe and affordable housing; dietary assistance through group meals and home meals; communications and transportation services; recreation and education opportunities; in-house services such as homemaker, visiting nurse and home health aides care; reading aids; and access to advice and services from appropriate health professionals.

APPENDIX II

SOURCES OF ADDITIONAL INFORMATION

Additional information about various health promotion and disease prevention activities is available from a number of sources. This section lists representative sources of information, grouped by the 15 activity areas introduced in Section III. Both government agencies and private, non-profit groups are listed. These agencies and organizations comprise only a portion of the total possible sources. Many other qualified sources of such information exist, including State and local health agencies which generally provide a comprehensive repository of consumer-oriented health information. Most groups listed offer free or low cost literature. The Surgeon General does not necessarily endorse the statements or viewpoints of the organizations listed.

PREVENTIVE HEALTH SERVICES

Family Planning

- *Planned Parenthood Federation of America, Inc.*
  810 Seventh Avenue
  New York, New York 10019
  (212) 541-7800

- *National Family Planning and Reproductive Health Association, Inc.*
  Suite 350
  425 Thirteenth Street, N.W.
  Washington, D.C. 20004
  (202) 783-1560

- *American College of Obstetricians and Gynecologists*
  Resource Center
  Suite 2700
  1 East Wacker Drive
  Chicago, Illinois 60601
  (312) 222-1600

- *National Clearinghouse for Family Planning Information*
  6110 Executive Blvd., Suite 250
  Rockville, Maryland 29852
  (301) 881-9400

Pregnancy and Infant Care

- *Office of Maternal and Child Health*
  Program Services Branch
  Bureau of Community Health Services
  Health Services Administration
  Room 7A20, Parklawn
  5600 Fishers Lane
  Rockville, Maryland 20857
  (301) 443-4273

- *National Foundation—March of Dimes*
  Public Health Education Department
  1275 Mamaroneck Avenue
  White Plains, New York 10605
  (914) 428-7100,

- *American College of Obstetricians and Gynecologists*
  Resource Center
  Suite 2700
  1 East Wacker Drive
  Chicago, Illinois 60601
  (312) 222-1600

- *American Academy of Pediatrics*
  1801 Hinman Avenue
  Evanston, Illinois 60204
  (312) 869-4255

Immunizations

- *Center for Disease Control*
  Bureau of State Services
  Technical Information Services
  Center for Disease Control
  Atlanta, Georgia 30333
  (404) 452-4021

- *National Institute of Child Health and Human Development*
  Office of Research Reporting
  Room 2A34, Building 31
  National Institutes of Health
  Bethesda, Maryland 20205
  (301) 496-5133

Sexually Transmissible Diseases

- *Center for Disease Control*
  Bureau of State Services
  Technical Information Services
  Center for Disease Control
  Atlanta, Georgia 30333
  (404) 452-4021

- *American Social Health Association*
  260 Sheridan Avenue
  Palo Alto, California 94306
  (415) 321-5134

- *VD National Hot Line*
  260 Sheridan Avenue
  Palo Alto, California 94306
  (800) 227-8922

High Blood Pressure and Heart Disease

- *National High Blood Pressure Information Center*
  Suite 1300
  7910 Woodmont Avenue
  Bethesda, Maryland 20014
  (301) 652-7700

- *National Heart, Lung, and Blood Institute*
  Public Inquiries Office
  Room 4A21, Building 31
  National Institutes of Health
  Bethesda, Maryland 20205
  (301) 496-4236

- *American Heart Association*
  7320 Greenville Avenue
  Dallas, Texas 75231
  (214) 750-5300
  (or local chapters)

- *Consumer Information Center*
  Consumer Information Center
  Pueblo, Colorado 81009
  (303) 544-5277, ext. 370

HEALTH PROTECTION

Toxic Agent Control

- *Center for Disease Control*
  Chronic Diseases Division
  Bureau of Epidemiology
  Building 1, Room 5127
  Center for Disease Control
  Atlanta, Georgia 30333
  (404) 329-3165

- *Environmental Protection Agency*
  Office of Public Awareness
  Environmental Protection Agency
  401 M Street, S.W.
  Mail Code: A-107
  Washington, D.C. 20460
  (202) 755-0700

- *National Institute of Environmental Health Sciences*
  National Institutes of Health
  Post Office Box 12233
  Research Triangle Park, North Carolina 27709
  (919) 541-3345

- *American Lung Association*
  1740 Broadway
  New York, New York 10019
  (212) 245-8000
  (or local chapter)

Occupational Safety and Health

- *Occupational Safety and Health Administration*
  Office of Public and Consumer Affairs
  U.S. Department of Labor (Room N3637)
  200 Constitution Avenue, N.W.
  Washington, D.C. 20210
  (202) 523-8151

- *Clearinghouse for Occupational Safety and Health*
  National Institute for Occupational Safety and Health
  Center for Disease Control
  Robert A. Taft Laboratory
  4676 Columbia Parkway
  Cincinnati, Ohio 45226
  (513) 684-8326

- *National Safety Council*
  444 North Michigan Avenue
  Chicago, Illinois 60611
  (312) 527-4800

- *American Industrial Hygiene Association*
  475 Wolf Ledges Parkway
  Akron, Ohio 44311
  (216) 762-7294

- *American Occupational Medical Association*
  Suite 2240
  150 North Wacker Drive
  Chicago, Illinois 60606
  (312) 782-2166

Accidental Injury Control

- *Consumer Product Safety Commission*
  Consumer Education and Awareness Division
  5401 Westbard Avenue
  Washington, D.C. 20207
  (202) 492-6576
  (or local Poison Control Centers)

- *Department of Transportation*
  General Services Division (NAD-42)
  National Highway Traffic Safety Administration
  Department of Transportation
  400 Seventh Street, S.W. (Room 4423)
  Washington, D.C. 20590
  (202) 426-0874
  ATTN: E. Kitts

- *National Safety Council*
  444 North Michigan Avenue
  Chicago, Illinois 60611
  (312) 527-4800

- *American Red Cross*
  National Headquarters
  18th and E Streets, N.W.
  Washington, D.C. 20006
  (202) 857-3555

Community Water Supply Fluoridation

- *Center for Disease Control*
  Dental Disease Prevention Activity (E107)
  Center for Disease Control
  Atlanta, Georgia 30333
  (404) 262-6631

- *National Institute of Dental Research*
  Public Inquiries Office
  Room 2C34, Building 31
  National Institutes of Health
  Bethesda, Maryland 20205
  (301) 496-4261

- *American Dental Association*
  Bureau of Health Education and Audiovisual Services
  American Dental Association
  211 East Chicago Avenue
  Chicago, Illinois 60611
  (312) 440-2593

Infectious Agent Control

- *Center for Disease Control*
  Public Inquiries
  Management Analysis and Service Office
  Building 4, Room B2
  Center for Disease Control
  Atlanta, Georgia 30333
  (404) 329-3534

- *National Institute of Allergy and Infectious Diseases*
  Office of Research Reporting and Public Response
  Room 7A32, Building 31
  National Institutes of Health
  Bethesda, Maryland 20205
  (301) 496-5717

HEALTH PROMOTION

Smoking Cessation

- *Technical Information Center for Smoking and Health*
  Office on Smoking and Health
  Department of Health, Education, and Welfare
  Room 1-16, Park Building
  5600 Fishers Lane
  Rockville, Maryland 20857
  (301) 443-1690

- *Office of Cancer Communications*
  National Cancer Institute
  Room 10A18, Building 31
  National Institutes of Health
  Bethesda, Maryland 20205
  (301) 496-5583

- *American Cancer Society*
  Public Information Department
  777 Third Avenue
  New York, New York 10017
  (212) 371-2900, ext. 254
  (or local chapter)

- *American Lung Association*
  1740 Broadway
  New York, New York 10019
  (212) 245-8000
  (or local chapter)

- *American Heart Association*
  7320 Greenville Avenue
  Dallas, Texas 75231
  (214) 750-5300
  (or local chapter)

Reducing Misuse of Alcohol and Drugs

- *National Clearinghouse on Alcohol Information*
  Post Office Box 2345
  Rockville, Maryland 20852
  (301) 468-2600

- *National Clearinghouse on Drug Abuse Information*
  Room 10A53, Parklawn Building
  5600 Fishers Lane
  Rockville, Maryland 20857
  (301) 443-6500

- *National Council on Alcoholism*
  733 Third Avenue
  New York, New York 10017
  (212) 986-4433

- *Alcoholics Anonymous*
  General Services Office (6th Floor)
  468 Park Avenue South
  New York, New York 10016
  (212) 686-1100
  ATTN: Public Information Department

Improved Nutrition

- *Food and Drug Administration*
  Office of Consumer Communications (HFG-10)
  Food and Drug Administration
  Room 15B32, Parklawn Building
  5600 Fishers Lane
  Rockville, Maryland 20857
  (301) 443-3170

- *U.S. Department of Agriculture*
  Human Nutrition Center SEA
  Room 421A
  U.S. Department of Agriculture
  Washington, D.C. 20250
  (202) 447-7854

- *Consumer Information Center*
  Consumer Information Center
  Pueblo, Colorado 81009
  (303) 544-5277, ext. 370

- *Nutrition Foundation*
  Suite 300
  888 Seventeenth Street, N.W.
  Washington, D.C. 20006
  (202) 872-0778

- *National Nutrition Education Clearinghouse*
    Suite 1110
    2140 Shattuck Avenue
    Berkeley, California 94704
    (415) 548-1363

Exercise and Fitness

- *President's Council on Physical Fitness and Sports*
    Department of Health, Education and Welfare
    Room 3030 Donohoe Building
    400 Sixth Street, S.W.
    Washington, D.C. 20201
    (202) 755-7947

- *American Alliance for Health, Physical Education, Recreation, and Dance*
    Promotions Unit
    1201 Sixteenth Street, N.W.
    Washington, D.C. 20036
    (202) 833-5534

- *American College of Sports Medicine*
    1440 Monroe Street
    Madison, Wisconsin 53706
    (608) 262-3632

Stress Control

- *National Clearinghouse for Mental Health Information*
    National Institute of Mental Health
    Room 11A33, Parklawn Building
    5600 Fishers Lane
    Rockville, Maryland 20857
    (301) 443-4517

- *Mental Health Association*
    1800 North Kent Street
    Arlington, Virginia 22209
    (or local chapters)
    (703) 528-6405

- *Public Affairs Committee, Inc.*
    Room 1101
    381 Park Avenue South
    New York, New York 10016
    (212) 683-4331

- *Blue Cross and Blue Shield Associations*
    Public Relations Office
    840 North Lake Shore Drive
    Chicago, Illinois 60611
    (312) 440-5955

GENERAL INFORMATION SOURCES

Public Health Service

- *Bureau of Health Education*
  Building 14
  Center for Disease Control
  Atlanta, Georgia 30333
  (404) 329-3111

- *Office of Health Information and Health Promotion*
  Office of the Surgeon General
  Department of Health, Education, and Welfare (Room 721B HHH)
  200 Independence Avenue, S.W.
  Washington, D.C.
  (202) 472-5370

National Organizations

- *National Association of Community Health Centers, Inc.*
  Suite 420
  1625 Eye Street, N.W.
  Washington, D.C. 20006
  (202) 833-9280

- *National Center for Health Education*
  211 Sutter Street (4th Floor)
  San Francisco, California 94108
  (415) 781-6144

State and Local Levels

- *Contact your family physician*
- *Contact your local health department*
- *Contact your county's cooperative extension service*

ACKNOWLEDGEMENTS

Preparation of this report was coordinated by the U.S. Public Health Service's Office of Disease Prevention and Health Promotion, directed by J. Michael McGinnis, M.D., Deputy Assistant Secretary for Health. Contributions were made by a wide variety of agencies and individuals, listed below. Special acknowledgement should be given to the Institute of Medicine of the National Academy of Sciences, which developed a series of scientific background papers for the report, as well as to the Center for Disease Control and the National Center for Health Statistics, which contributed substantially to the development of the data and tables contained in the report.

PARTICIPATING AGENCIES

The following Federal agencies contributed to preparation and review of the report:

Public Health Service (HEW)

Alcohol, Drug Abuse, and Mental Health Administration
Gerald L. Klerman, M.D., Administrator

Center for Disease Control
William H. Foege, M.D., Director

Food and Drug Administration
Donald Kennedy, Ph.D., Commissioner

Health Resources Administration
Henry A. Foley, Ph.D., Administrator

Health Services Administration
George I. Lythcott, M.D., Administrator

National Center for Health Statistics
Dorothy P. Rice, Director

National Institutes of Health
Donald S. Fredrickson, M.D., Director

Office of Health Planning and Evaluation
James Mongan, M.D., Deputy Assistant Secretary for Health

Office of Population Affairs
Irvin M. Cushner, M.D., Deputy Assistant Secretary for Health

Office of Public Affairs
Michael F. White, Director

Office of Research, Statistics and Technology
Ruth S. Hanft, Deputy Assistant Secretary for Health

Office on Smoking and Health
John M. Pinney, Director

Department of Agriculture

M. Rupert Cutler, Ph.D.
Assistant Secretary for Conservation, Research and Education

Carol Tucker Foreman
Assistant Secretary for Food and Consumer Services

Department of Labor

Eula Bingham, Ph.D.
Assistant Secretary for Occupational Safety and Health

Department of Transportation

Joan Claybrook, Administrator
National Highway Traffic Safety Administration

Department of the Treasury

Richard J. Davis
Assistant Secretary for Enforcement and Operations

Consumer Product Safety Commission

Susan B. King, Chairman

Environmental Protection Agency

Douglas M. Costle, Administrator

CONTRIBUTORS

The following individuals contributed materials to the development of the manuscript:

Irwin L. Auerbach, Program Analyst, Environmental Protection Agency

Norman W. Axnick, Director, Office of Program Planning and Evaluation, Center for Disease Control, U.S. Public Health Service

Clement Barbaza, Printing and Reproduction Management Branch Chief, Office of Management, Office of the Assistant Secretary for Health, U.S. Public Health Service (production assistance)

Katharine Bauer, Senior Advisor, Office of Health Information, Health Promotion and Physical Fitness and Sports Medicine, U.S. Public Health Service

Alexander Cohen, Ph.D., Chief, Behavioral and Motivational Factors Branch, Division of Biomedical and Behavioral Science, National Institute for Occupational Safety and Health, Center for Disease Control, U.S. Public Health Service

Ralph Cosham, Editorial Consultant, Office of Health Information, Health Promotion and Physical Fitness and Sports Medicine, U.S. Public Health Service

Audrey T. Cross, Nutrition Policy Coordinator, Office of the Secretary, U.S. Department of Agriculture

Paul Danaceau, Editorial Consultant, Office of Disease Prevention and Health Promotion, U.S. Public Health Service

Winthrop N. Davey, M.D., Director, Bureau of Training, Center for Disease Control, U.S. Public Health Service

Ervin S. Duggan, Special Assistant to the Secretary, Department of Health, Education, and Welfare

Lawrence Farer, M.D., Director, Tuberculosis Division, Bureau of State Services, Center for Disease Control, U.S. Public Health Service

Barry Felrice, Acting Associate Administrator for Plans and Programs, National Highway Traffic Safety Administration, Department of Transportation

Allen Forbes, M.D., Director, Nutrition and Consumer Sciences, Food and Drug Administration, U.S. Public Health Service

David Fraser, M.D., Chief, Special Pathogens Branch, Bacterial Diseases Division, Bureau of Epidemiology, Center for Disease Control, U.S. Public Health Service

Frank Frodyma, Operations Research Analyst, Occupational Safety and Health Administration, Department of Labor

Lawrence Galton, Editorial Consultant, Office of Disease Prevention and Health Promotion, U.S. Public Health Service

John C. Greene, D.M.D., Deputy Surgeon General, U.S. Public Health Service

Michael B. Gregg, M.D., Deputy Director, Bureau of Epidemiology, Center for Disease Control, U.S. Public Health Service

Stephen W. Havas, M.D., Medical Advisor, Office of Health Information, Health Promotion and Physical Fitness and Sports Medicine, U.S. Public Health Service

John W. Horm, Statistician, Demographic Analysis Section, Biometry Branch, National Cancer Institute, National Institutes of Health, U.S. Public Health Service

Juel Janis, Ph.D., Special Assistant to the Assistant Secretary for Health and Surgeon General, U.S. Public Health Service

John T. Kalberer, Jr., Ph.D., Assistant Director, Office for Medical Applications of Research, National Institutes of Health, U.S. Public Health Service

Vicki Kalmar, Professional Associate, Division of Health Promotion and Disease Prevention, The Institute of Medicine, National Academy of Sciences

Martha Katz, Special Assistant to the Deputy Assistant Secretary for Health, Office of Disease Prevention and Health Promotion, U.S. Public Health Service

Samuel S. Kessel, M.D., Robert Wood Johnson Foundation Fellow, Office of the Assistant Secretary for Health, U.S. Public Health Service

Ronald J. Kostraba, Technical Services Specialist, Administrative Services Center, Office of Management, Office of the Assistant Secretary for Health, U.S. Public Health Service (cover design)

J. Michael Lane, M.D., Director, Bureau of Smallpox Eradication, Center for Disease Control, U.S. Public Health Service

Seth N. Leibler, Ed.D., Deputy Director, Bureau of Training, Center for Disease Control, U.S. Public Health Service

Frank S. Lisella, Ph.D., Program Development Branch, Environmental Health Services Division, Bureau of State Services, Center for Disease Control, U.S. Public Health Service

Brian J. McCarthy, M.D., Family Planning Evaluation Division, Bureau of Epidemiology, Center for Disease Control, U.S. Public Health Service

J. Donald Millar, M.D., Director, Bureau of State Services, Center for Disease Control, U.S. Public Health Service

Sanford Miller, Ph.D., Director, Bureau of Foods, Food and Drug Administration, U.S. Public Health Service

Catherine Milton, Special Assistant to the Assistant Secretary for Enforcement and Operations, Department of the Treasury

John E. Mounts, Publications Branch Chief, National Center for Health Satistics, U.S. Public Health Service

Elena O. Nightingale, M.D., Ph.D., Director, Division of Health Promotion and Disease Prevention, The Institute of Medicine, National Academy of Sciences

Godfrey P. Oakley, Jr., M.D., Chief, Birth Defects Branch, Chronic Diseases Division, Bureau of Epidemiology, Center for Disease Control, U.S. Public Health Service

Horace G. Ogden, Director, Bureau of Health Education, Center for Disease Control, U.S. Public Health Service

Jennifer Peck, Social Science Analyst, Bureau of the Census, Department of Commerce

Earl S. Pollock, Sc.D., Chief, Biometry Branch, National Cancer Institute, National Institutes of Health, U.S. Public Health Service

Thomas W. Poore, Chief, Text Preparation Section, Publications Branch, National Center for Health Statistics, U.S. Public Health Service

Kate Prager, Sc.D., Statistician, Mortality Statistics Branch, Division of Vital Statistics, National Center for Health Statistics, U.S. Public Health Service

Robert Proctor, Public Affairs Officer, Office of Public Affairs, U.S. Public Health Service

David Rall, M.D., Director, National Institute of Environmental Health Sciences, National Institutes of Health, U.S. Public Health Service

Robert L. Ringler, Ph.D., Deputy Director, National Institute on Aging, National Institutes of Health, U.S. Public Health Service

Don Robinson, Printing Specialist, Printing and Reproduction Management Branch, Office of Management, Office of the Assistant Secretary for Health, U.S. Public Health Service (production assistance)

Harry Rosenberg, Ph.D., Chief, Mortality Statistics Branch, Division of Vital Statistics, National Center for Health Statistics, U.S. Public Health Service

Lisbeth Bamberger Schorr, Chairperson, Select Panel for the Promotion of Child Health

171

Roger Sherwin, M.D. Associate Professor, Department of Epidemiology and Preventive Medicine, University of Maryland

Michael Smith, Ph.D., Chief, Motivational and Stress Research Section, Behavioral and Motivational Factors Branch, National Institute for Occupational Safety and Health, Center for Disease Control, U.S. Public Health Service

James W. Stratton, M.D., Medical Officer/Prevention Planning, Office of Program Planning and Evaluation, Center for Disease Control, U.S. Public Health Service

Ronald D. Teske, Health Analysis and Planning for Preventive Services, Bureau of State Services, Center for Disease Control, U.S. Public Health Service

Susan B. Toal, M.P.H., Instructional Systems Specialist, Bureau of Training, Center for Disease Control, U.S. Public Health Service

Dennis D. Tolsma, M.P.H., Program Analysis Officer, Office of Program Planning and Evaluation, Center for Disease Control, U.S. Public Health Service

Carl W. Tyler, M.D., Director, Family Planning Evaluation Division, Bureau of Epidemiology, Center for Disease Control, U.S. Public Health Service

Daniel C. VanderMeer, Project Manager, Childhood Immunization Initiative, U.S. Public Health Service

William Walton, III, Acting Director, Office of Strategic Planning, Consumer Product Safety Commission

Basil Whiting, Deputy Assistant Secretary, Occupational Safety and Health Administration, Department of Labor

Ronald W. Wilson, Chief, Health Status and Demographic Analysis Branch, Division of Analysis, National Center for Health Statistics, U.S. Public Health Service

David Wu, Program Analyst, Office of Health Information, Health Promotion and Physical Fitness and Sports Medicine, U.S. Public Health Service

REVIEWERS

The following individuals provided review and comments for the development of the manuscript:

Herbert K. Abrams, M.D., M.P.H., Director of the Arizona Center for Occupational Safety and Health, Arizona Health Sciences Center, University of Arizona

Duane Alexander, M.D., Assistant to the Director, National Institute of Child Health and Human Development, National Institutes of Health, U.S. Public Health Service

John R. Ball, M.D., J.D., Senior Policy Analyst, Office of Science and Technology Policy, Executive Office of the President

Robert Benedict, Commissioner, Administration on Aging, Office of Human Development Services

Christopher Bladen, Director, Division of Health Evaluation and Prevention, Office of the Assistant Secretary for Planning and Evaluation/ Health, Department of Health, Education, and Welfare

Martha Blaxall, Acting Director, Office of Research, Health Care Financing Administration

George A. Bray, M.D., Nutrition Coordinator, U.S. Public Health Service

Lester Breslow, M.D., M.P.H., Dean, School of Public Health, Center for the Health Sciences, University of California at Los Angeles

John H. Bryant, M.D., Deputy Assistant Secretary for International Health, U.S. Public Health Service

Benjamin T. Burton, Ph.D., Associate Director, National Institute of Arthritis, Metabolism, and Digestive Diseases, National Institutes of Health, U.S. Public Health Service

Kathy Buto, Policy Coordinator, Executive Secretariat, Office of the Secretary, Department of Health, Education, and Welfare

C. Carson Conrad, Executive Director, President's Council on Physical Fitness and Sports, U.S. Public Health Service

Richard Cotton, Executive Secretary, Department of Health, Education, and Welfare

Charles L. Cox, Assistant to the Director of the Bureau of Radiological Health, Food and Drug Administration, U.S. Public Health Service

Lawrence R. Deyton, Public Health Analyst, Office of Program Development, Office of Health Research, Statistics, and Technology, U.S. Public Health Service

James F. Dickson, III, M.D., Senior Advisor for Environmental Affairs, U.S. Public Health Service

Ronald Dobbin, M.Sc. Industrial Hygiene Engineer, National Institute for Occupational Safety and Health, Center for Disease Control, U.S. Public Health Service

Allen Duncan, Assistant for Program Operations, Office of Health Affairs, Food and Drug Administration, U.S. Public Health Service

Jack Elinson, Ph.D., Service Fellow, Division of Analysis, National Center for Health Statistics, U.S. Public Health Service

Manning Feinleib, M.D., Dr. P.H., Acting Director of Epidemiology and Biometry, National Heart, Lung, and Blood Institute, National Institute of Health, U.S. Public Health Service

Jacob J. Feldman, Ph.D., Associate Director for Analysis, National Center for Health Statistics, U.S. Public Health Service

Kenneth Flieger, Special Assistant to the Acting Associate Commissioner for Health Affairs, Food and Drug Administration, U.S. Public Health Service

Calvin Frederick, Ph.D., Chief, Disaster Assistance and Emergency Mental Health Section, Division of Special Mental Health Programs, National Institute of Mental Health, Alcohol, Drug Abuse, and Mental Health Administration, U.S. Public Health Service

Terry Freeman, Clearinghouse Coordinator, Office of Health Information, Health Promotion and Physical Fitness and Sports Medicine, U.S. Public Health Service

Peter L. Frommer, M.D., Deputy Director, National Heart, Lung, and Blood Institute, National Institutes of Health, U.S. Public Health Service

Carol W. Garvey, M.D., Acting Chief Medical Officer, Office of Primary Care, Bureau of Community Health Services, Health Services Administration, U.S. Public Health Service

Stephen E. Goldston, Ed.D., M.S.P.H., Coordinator for Primary Prevention Programs, National Institute of Mental Health, Alcohol, Drug Abuse, and Mental Health Administration, U.S. Public Health Service

David A. Hamburg, M.D., President, The Institute of Medicine, National Academy of Sciences

Stephen P. Hersh, M.D., Assistant Director for Children and Youth, National Institute of Mental Health, Alcohol, Drug Abuse, and Mental Health Administration, U.S. Public Health Service

174

Richard N. Hill, Acting Director, Health Effects and Science Policy, Office of Toxic Substances, Environmental Protection Agency

Donald R. Hopkins, M.D. Assistant Director for International Health, Center for Disease Control, U.S. Public Health Service

Mary Jane Jesse, M.D., Director, Division of Heart and Vascular Diseases, National Heart, Lung, and Blood Institute, National Institutes of Health, U.S. Public Health Service

Joel Kavet, Associate Director for Program Development, Office of Health Research, Statistics, and Technology, U.S. Public Health Service

Miller H. Kerr, Planning and Evaluation, Bureau of State Services, Center for Disease Control, U.S. Public Health Service

George M. Kingman, Director, Office of Program Planning and Evaluation, National Institute of Environmental Health Sciences, National Institutes of Health, U.S. Public Health Service

Charles Krauthammer, M.D., Special Assistant to the Administrator, Alcohol, Drug Abuse, and Mental Health Administration, U.S. Public Health Service

George A. Lamb, M.D., Associate Professor, Department of Preventive and Social Medicine, Harvard Medical School

Mildred K. Lehman, Director, Office of Communications and Public Affairs, Alcohol, Drug Abuse, and Mental Health Administration, U.S. Public Health Service

Mark H. Lepper, M.D., Vice-President of Evaluation, Rush Medical Center, Chicago, Illinois

Charles U. Lowe, M.D., Director, Office of Child Health Affairs, U.S. Public Health Service

Bernard R. McColgan, Chief, Prevention Branch, National Institute on Drug Abuse, Alcohol, Drug Abuse, and Mental Health Administration, U.S. Public Health Service

Carolyn G. McHale, Head, Program Information Section, National Eye Institute, National Institutes of Health, U.S. Public Health Service

Laura A. Miller, Special Assistant to the Secretary, Department of Health, Education, and Welfare

Lulu Mae Nix, Ed.D., Director, Office of Adolescent Pregnancy Programs, Office of the Assistant Secretary for Health, U.S. Public Health Service

Mark Novitch, M.D., Acting Associate Commissioner for Health Affairs, Food and Drug Administration, U.S. Public Health Service

Gilbert S. Omenn, M.D., Ph.D., Associate Director for Human Resources and Social and Economic Services, Office of Science and Technology Policy, Executive Office of the President

Seymour Perry, M.D., Associate Director for Medical Applications of Research, National Institutes of Health, U.S. Public Health Service

Blandina Ramirez, M.D., Commissioner, Administration for Children, Youth and Families, Office of Human Development Services

Roger W. Rochat, M.D., Deputy Director, Family Planning Evaluation Division, Bureau of Epidemiology, Center for Disease Control, U.S. Public Health Service

Renie Schapiro, M.P.H., Staff Fellow, Office of Health Affairs, Food and Drug Administration, U.S. Public Health Service

Marvin Schneiderman, Ph.D., Associate Director for Science Policy, National Cancer Institute, National Institutes of Health, U.S. Public Health Service

John R. Seal, M.D., Deputy Director, National Institute of Allergy and Infectious Diseases, National Institutes of Health, U.S. Public Health Service

Eva Sereghy, Media Coordinator, Office of Health Information, Health Promotion and Physical Fitness and Sports Medicine, U.S. Public Health Service

Cliff Sessions, Deputy Assistant Secretary for Public Affairs, Department of Health, Education, and Welfare

Zekin Shakhashiri, M.D., Special Assistant to the Chief, Office of Program Planning and Evaluation, National Institute of Neurological and Communicative Disorders and Stroke, U.S. Public Health Service

Laurel C. Shannon, Special Assistant to the Associate Administrator for Planning, Evaluation, and Legislation, Health Resources Administration, U.S. Public Health Service

L. David Taylor, Deputy Assistant Secretary for Management Analysis and Systems, Office of the Secretary, Department of Health, Education, and Welfare

Geraldine Tompkins, Social Science Specialist, Office of Health Information, Health Promotion and Physical Fitness and Sports Medicine, U.S. Public Health Service

Lyman Van Nostrand, Director, Division of Planning, Office of Planning, Evaluation, and Legislation, Health Resources Administration, U.S. Public Health Service

Howard R. Veit, Director, Office of Health Maintenance Organizations, Office of the Assistant Secretary for Health, U.S. Public Health Service

Graham W. Ward, M.P.H., Chief, Health Education Branch, Office of Prevention, Education, and Control, National Heart, Lung, and Blood Institute, National Institutes of Health, U.S. Public Health Service

Lois G. Whitley, Deputy Director, Division of Prevention, National Institute on Alcohol Abuse and Alcoholism, Alcohol, Drug Abuse, and Mental Health Administration, U.S. Public Health Service

Sidney C. Wolverton, Acting Associate Administrator for Program Coordination, Alcohol, Drug Abuse, and Mental Health Administration, U.S. Public Health Service

Matthew M. Zack, Jr., M.D., M.P.H., Cancer Branch, Chronic Diseases Division, Bureau of Epidemiology, Center for Disease Control, U.S. Public Health Service